INTRODUCTION
TO PALEO

Discover How to Lose Weight Today and Keep it off Forever

REBECCA FIELD

Published by Starfish Publishing UK

Copyright © Rebecca Field

Printed and bound in the UK by CMP (UK) Limited

First published in the UK 2015

A catalogue reference for this book is available
at the British Library

ISBN 978-0-9932593-0-2

Acknowledgments

To my husband, without you none of this would be possible.
I can never thank you enough for letting my dream become a reality.

To Anna whose passion and belief in the project has never wavered.

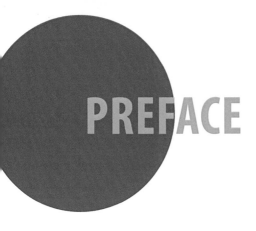

PREFACE

Before you start to read this book I wanted to give you an insight into my life so you can appreciate where the inspiration and passion has come from. Let's start at the beginning; my name is Rebecca Field and I am a reformed serial dieter.

The Dieting Years.....

My emotional relationship with food goes back as far as I can remember. It has been my reward for the good times and my emotional crutch through the bad times. Which one resulted in causing the most damage is hard to tell! It seems that there was never really a good reason as to why I should not be able to treat myself with food. It seemed only fair; everyone else was able to eat what they wanted to and not have to worry. Why not me? The problem is I am 5 foot 2 inches tall and can put weight on by just looking at a piece of cake. Combine this with my appetite, which can rival that of any rugby player, and it was never going to end well.

The result has been a lifetime of self-loathing followed by sporadic diets which were always going to be "the one" to change my life for good. Of course, they would all work for a while but inevitably, I would end up piling the weight back on (and then some!) and before long I would be back to square one. I have been a size 8 and I have been a size 16 as well as every possible size inbetween at least once. Over the years I learnt to perfect a happy face whilst I would try not to cry as I squeeze into my clothes, hating every single inch of my body and loathing myself for what I have let happen to myself…again. That question would always go through my mind, how have I done this to myself again? The answer of course was never forthcoming and I looked for it really hard; usually at the bottom of a family sized packet of crisps.

It's not that I don't have the determination to diet. I am one of the most stubborn people I know and once I set my mind to something I will make it happen (in fact this book itself is a result of such determination). I can't say it was all fat days and tears. I have had many "successful" diets along the way. These allowed me to experience the sheer delight of being able to walk with such pride and confidence in that pair of jeans which would linger at the back of the wardrobe usually only ventured to after a bout of food poisoning. That feeling I cannot deny is amazing. It makes you want to skip down the street and hug complete strangers. So where does it all go wrong?

The problem for me has always been maintaining my weight loss. Once I get to a certain point I just slip back into old ways. Then I utter the immortal words of "best to start the diet on Monday". Whilst this might sound rational to some people, this decision was inevitably made on a Tuesday afternoon after devouring a chocolate bar (and the rest) and then deciding "best to get it all out my system this week". The result would be an almighty binge of anything I could get my hands on. I don't think half the time I even wanted what I was eating. It was more a case of being "allowed" to eat it this week so best "fill my boots" before the next diet starts. The problem is the diet never did start on Monday.

I am still ashamed, even now, of my behaviour in the "bingeing" phases. I truly believe it is an addiction. I would fixate on food for my every waking moment and get agitated and distressed if I was challenged on my eating habits. The words "do you really think you should be eating that" would send me into an emotional frenzy. To avoid such confrontation, I would create situations whereby I could eat food on my own – away from those who knew me – away from judgment. I would despise myself afterwards, but very rarely could I ever stop myself. I dread to think what damage this cycle has caused to my body both emotionally and physically.

The Turning Point....

It was early 2009, I was living in Leeds and working as a Solicitor. I was having a fantastic time enjoying myself but this of course meant a lot of eating and drinking. The social aspect was practically part of the job description and I was having a great time.

However, the inevitable happened and I started to put weight on…yet again. After the usual crying, self-loathing and questioning as to how this had happened, I came to realise that, on the most practical level, I just couldn't afford to buy new suits every time I put weight on. I knew that I had to try and address the issue once and for all. I wanted to be professional and respected, which to me equated to getting a control of my weight issues. There was something inside of me that just knew I needed to make a change for the better.

I decided that I couldn't do it on my own; I needed some professional help. So I found a personal trainer. His name was Alan and without a doubt he changed my life. I won't pretend it happened overnight or that it was an easy process. In fact, to begin with I still seemed to be my own worst enemy. After seeing Alan for a couple of times a week for a few months he sat me down and we had a chat about what I really wanted to get out of the sessions. The problem was I was still eating and drinking too much and this was impacting on what benefit I could realistically get out of the training sessions. It really brought it home to me that if I wanted my life to change, I needed to commit.

The next day I heard from a friend who asked if I wanted to go on a villa holiday to France. Usually this would have filled me with fear as all I would be able to think about would be wearing a bikini in front of a large group of people. This time it all seemed to click. This could be my goal. I contacted Alan straight away and told him I was ready to commit. His response – this is the best decision you will ever make.

The Diet....

My next training session was spent discussing my new plan. Alan introduced me to the Paleo diet; we talked at length about what it would involve and the benefits that it would have for both my health and assisting with the training programme. It was explained to me that what I consumed was going to have the biggest impact on my body shape and wellbeing, and that no amount of exercise would get me there if I didn't commit to providing the best nourishment for my body.

I had strangely never associated any "diet" with actually providing nourishment to my body. It was usually just all about the weight loss and how I would look. I never previously considered that it would be beneficial to actively nourish my body. To me diets had always just been about that number on the scales, I had never given too much thought about how I should feel, or what I was doing to my body. I always just thought that a thin body had to equate to a healthier body right?

The first thing that struck me about the Paleo diet was that there was no calorie counting. The second was that you could eat foods high in "fats" (of course these are good fats) and the third was that I would not need to eat starchy carbs in order to provide fuel for my body. All of these were complete revelations to me and went against everything that I have ever believed I had known about "dieting". It turns out that, despite being a serial dieter, I knew shockingly little about what my body needed in order to function and how best to achieve that. The thing about the Paleo diet is that it is not really a "diet" at all but a way of allowing your body to function effectively and thereby shedding the excess weight is almost a side effect. In order to embrace this I needed to relearn everything that I thought I knew about dieting. It was long overdue!

The 12 Week Plan....

The first step was to re-educate myself, not only about food, but about my body and try to understand why I was eating. I kept a food diary for the first couple of weeks. Every time I ate I made a note of what I was eating, how I was feeling and whether I was craving any particular foods. I would strongly encourage everyone to do the same. When you have to actually sit down and listen to your body and think what it is you want and why it is quite eye opening.

From carrying out this exercise it was clear that my body was adjusting quickly to the Paleo diet. Any cravings that I had went after the first week and the comments about how I was feeling changed from "tired" "hungry" or "bored" to "energised" "excited" and "happy". I was shocked that I could actually physically feel the beneficial effects of the food that I was eating. Even better, I was really enjoying the food and never felt deprived. I loved not having to count calories.

I was practically bouncing off the walls with energy and was getting stronger and faster in the gym. I developed a profound clarity of mind, everything was much clearer and I no longer experienced any "head fogs" as I used to call them. I was sleeping much better and was more productive at work and most importantly, I was looking great. My body was changing shape, creating a longer leaner silhouette. I was full of energy, my skin was glowing and I felt confident - and this was only a couple of weeks in.

Of course there were changes that I had to make to my lifestyle. The biggest one was cutting back on drinking and eating out. This inevitably meant changing the structure of my social life. I won't lie to you and say this was easy. Nothing worth pursuing ever is. However, I knew deep down that if I wanted to change my lifestyle for the better, the socialising had to, at least at the beginning, take a hit. This didn't mean that I sat at home and failed to see anyone for months! I just had to learn to adapt my social life around what I was trying to achieve. I still saw my friends all the time and even had the occasional night out – it just made me realise how much better I felt when I didn't drink!

That is the great thing about the Paleo diet; it is all about finding the right balance for you. Once you have initially been able to adjust your body and lifestyle to the Paleo diet you can then clearly review and assess what will work best for you. You can integrate some foods back in if you wish to do so; it's all about finding that healthy balance. It is what makes it a lifestyle rather than a "diet" and is the reason that it is so successful at providing long lasting results.

By the time I reached the end of my 12 week programme my body fat had reduced by 16% and I was now on the border of ideal/lean on the body fat charts. I had lost well over a stone in weight and had converted a further stone of fat to lean muscle. For the first time in my life I was proud of my body. Not only had my body physically changed beyond recognition, but my outlook on life and approach to my health had been converted. I no longer assessed my health by the number showing on the scales nor do I fixate about my dress size. These things are no longer important to me. What is important is how I feel and how my body functions. I have learnt that once these are aligned the rest takes care of itself.

My Paleo journey started 5 years ago, and I have not looked back since. Whereas my usual approach to dieting would be to slowly revert back to old habits at the end of the "diet period" I found that my desire to continue with the Paleo diet was stronger than ever at the end of my 12 week programme.

I could not believe the results that I had achieved. They were truly incredible. I went on my villa holiday to France a completely changed person. My friends and family could not believe what I had achieved in such a short period of time. However, the best thing about the holiday turned out not to be wearing a bikini with pride – but meeting my now husband. This felt like the ultimate reward for all my hard work.

The Paleo Years....

So where am I now? Well, after meeting my husband in France the only problem was that he lived in London. So I moved to London in May 2010 and we got married in December 2012. I continued in my career as a Solicitor until early 2014 when I decided that it wasn't the long term career I wanted. Having spent the majority of my working life in a high stress, demanding and, quite frankly, soul destroying environment, I decided that I wanted to take control of my life and do something I enjoyed. After all, life is too short to think about the "what ifs".

When I thought about the things I was passionate about in life there was one thing that kept coming up over and over again – diet and fitness. It has, in one way or another, been such a big part of my life for as long as I can remember. The more I thought about it, the more it made sense. I really wanted to help others to achieve the transformation from a serial dieter to a healthy sustainable lifestyle - and that is why Paleo Diet and Fitness was created.

To create the Paleo Diet and Fitness eBooks, I have worked very closely with diet, nutrition and exercise professionals in order to provide the highest quality information and advice on the Paleo diet. From my own personal experience, I wanted to emphasise the importance of both diet and fitness in order to create a sustainable new lifestyle. I therefore wanted to create a programme which provided all the information you would need to start your own Paleo journey.

I am positive that you will find great success and a healthier life through following my Paleo Diet and Fitness Plan. I wish you the best of luck.

Embrace the power of Paleo and don't look back.

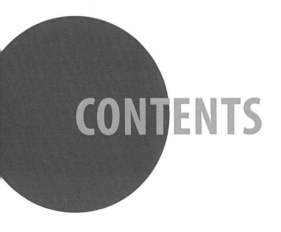

CONTENTS

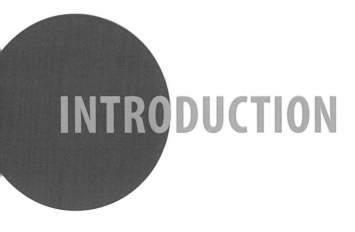

INTRODUCTION

The chances are that you have tried many approaches to weight loss and found that they have not been right for you. You may have initially lost weight but found the regime too difficult to follow, or you may have had complete success only to see the weight eventually return; even if you continued to follow the healthy eating guidelines. Gaining weight, for most of us, is exceptionally easy; losing it may be one of the hardest of life's obstacles that you ever have to face. Being overweight or obese is not only life threatening but can be a constant source of low self-esteem, disillusionment and even embarrassment; however convincing your happy face may be.

The Paleo lifestyle is fast becoming one of the most adopted ways of eating in the modern world. Increasing evidence shows that our industrial diet is harming not only our health but also that of the world in which we live; in fact, more and more people are beginning to question the way that they eat. With a focus on natural ingredients and whole foods, Paleo supports this drive towards real food, giving us back control over what we eat and encouraging us to regain the cooking skills that are all but lost.

Our Paleo plan has been designed to help you transform every aspect of your health and wellbeing to achieve a sustainable and healthy lifestyle. A whole body approach is central to the Paleo ethos and we embrace this wholeheartedly with plenty of ideas to keep your body active and mind relaxed. We therefore recommend that Introduction to Paleo is used in conjunction with Tabata Transformation, Introduction to Yoga and Paleo: 12 Weeks to Change Your Life.

Our interpretation of the Paleo diet is one that brings the latest thinking in nutrition together with techniques in self-development and coaching. We are aware that not everybody is a dedicated athlete or health-nut and that most people are actually quite fond of doughnuts. Modern living can be stressful, with jobs that aren't ideal and ends that barely meet, but by learning to take control of your food you will equip yourself with the tools needed to not only finally lose the weight, but to face life head on and with a spring in your spritely new step.

Introduction to Paleo will guide you through the concept that is Paleo. We show you what happens to the food that enters your body and why previous attempts at weight loss may have failed. Current thinking on fat, sugar and carbohydrate are examined closely so that you may gain a better understanding of why you so often feel powerless in the face of food.

We provide a 7 day recipe plan which is full of delicious food as well as tips for wellbeing and preparation. This will get you off to the great start that you need and introduce you to the Paleo way of eating. The recipes are all simple to cook and designed to provide you with what you may need most at every step of this initial stage. Once you have completed your first week *Paleo: 12 Weeks to Change Your Life* will take you through everything that you need to know to make that transition to a truly healthy and sustainable lifestyle that you can maintain forever.

Treating this Paleo reset as a holistic journey is an important part of success. Knowing and understanding yourself, as well as the processes within, are the keys to effective lifelong change. Looking at your life in terms of managing stress, getting adequate exercise, and promoting quality sleep form a solid base from which to explore the possibilities of a healthy and happy life.

Sound good? Then get ready to take control.

SECTION 1
What is the Paleo Diet?

The Paleo diet sprang from a growing body of research and evidence that suggests our Neolithic forefathers were at the peak of their physical and mental wellbeing and that this was due largely to their diet. This is why the Paleo diet is often referred to as "The Caveman Diet".

Human life was originally nomadic, with a diet made up of foods that could be hunted and gathered. As populations grew, and humans began to settle, the diet changed to consist of foods that could be grown or raised. We eventually ended up dwelling in large cities, far removed from the food that we eat and largely dependent upon industrial agriculture and processing for our daily nourishment. Early farming marked the beginning of growing cereal crops for food; a cheap food that is in practically everything we eat (whether we asked for it or not) and also feeds the intensively farmed livestock that we eat for meat.

Our health, despite so many advances that have seen off the fatal epidemics of earlier times, has never been as bad as it is today and the world's economy, and therefore healthcare services, are suffering for it. We see a pattern of malaise, aging debilitation and chronic illness that continues to rise. Many of us are physically unfit, dependant on prescription medication or just plain exhausted. Heart disease, cancer and diabetes are the killers of our time. Fewer people are leaving home with the cookery and home economics skills that are vital to the health of ours and future generations; this leaves the floor wide open for dependence on processed foods.

My job meant that I had to continually rely on processed convenience food and I was hardly ever at home to cook. The times when I did make it home at a reasonable hour (quite sadly this would still be after 9pm) all I could manage was a microwave meal and a packet of biscuits. It never occurred to me that if I took time to nourish my body that I would start to feel less tired and lethargic. Within just a few days of starting the Paleo diet I could not believe the difference that cutting out the processed food made to my energy levels. After a few weeks my eczema had practically gone and my skin was glowing. I could also think much clearer and those late nights became less painful and more productive.

The bedrock of the Paleo diet is REAL food. It firmly believes that a diet of meat, fish and plants is the way to optimum health. Some of the foods that Paleo excludes are the key to your weight loss, whilst others are more about fine tuning health; the further you explore the connection between food and your body it becomes clear that the two are not mutually exclusive. Essentially, Paleo is about eating clean; a phrase that crops up within various whole foods arenas that simply means to avoid all processed industrial foods and eat a diet of healthy produce. Once you have followed a Paleo lifestyle for a while you will identify with this term strongly. Your body will feel unencumbered by toxins and inflammation but should you decide to eat something processed or highly refined then the feeling is definitely one of needing to "re-cleanse".

Paleo believes that many of the foods we view as healthy can actually be harmful to our health and affect weight loss in ways that you may never even have considered. The current medical model of a healthy diet is under fire from new research; based as it is upon directives that are almost half a century old, a growing number of people are seriously beginning to question, and even disprove, its logic.

We are going to expand upon this and show you exactly how Paleo can help you to lose weight for life.

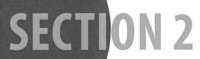

SECTION 2

How can Paleo help me lose weight when other diets have failed?

The key theme of modern weight loss management is the fact that you will only lose weight if you use more calories than you consume. Whilst this is an immutable physical fact, it is also true that the body does not use all calories in the same way and therefore there must be deeper underlying mechanisms involved. Put this together with the fact that food manufacturers, doctors and nutritionists have been pushing a high-carb, low-fat diet for the past fifty years and you can begin to see why so many individuals are starting to question a rationale that could well be responsible for the world's greatest obesity epidemic.

As you will see as you progress through Introduction to Paleo, until your diet addresses your delicate hormonal balance and looks at the body as a whole person functioning within an increasingly toxic environment then weight loss will be difficult to achieve and even harder to maintain. The word diet may have become synonymous with restrictive eating plans focused purely on the goal of losing weight but it actually stems from classical languages and means "way of life".

The foods that you eat drive your eating behaviour

When it comes down to it, your body exists as a series of reactions at the molecular level. These complex biochemical mechanisms drive not only your physical reactions but are responsible for your behaviour too. Body and brain are intricately interconnected; understanding this may be the key that you need to finally conquer your weight loss.

By following a Paleo eating plan you will reset your entire biochemical system and regain control over your body. You may believe it is greed that drives you to the bottom of the biscuit packet; it isn't. Your body and your brain are simply responding to a complex system of messages that has gone awry; the messages are muddled and can no longer communicate effectively. Your body is telling you to eat food that you do not need or even want. Food is there to heal not harm but, with your body stuck in a cycle of self-destruction, the path to wellness becomes unclear. Let's take a closer look at how this works.

As you progress through your Paleo journey you will start to notice very quickly how your approach to food and your body changes. I was amazed at how my cravings would disappear and that the desire to continually overeat could be overcome so easily. In fact, I have never felt as full as when I started my Paleo journey. I didn't feel deprived or restricted and was looking forward to every meal.

Insulin is everything

It largely revolves around insulin. Most of us are aware that insulin has something to do with blood sugar and is relevant to those with diabetes. You may be familiar with the concept of GI foods and glycaemic load; scales of measurement that inform us how much carbohydrate a food contains and how likely it is to affect our blood sugar.

But have you ever considered just how much your weight loss efforts are dominated by the insulin in your body?

Grasp this one fact and you will finally learn, and understand, not only how to lose weight effectively but how to keep it off for life. Insulin, hormonal balance and human metabolism are complex mechanisms that science is still working hard to fathom completely but great leaps and strides have been made in recent years that give us much better insight. These complex mechanisms work in minute synchronicity with each other and there are other important aspects to consider when battling against weight gain that we shall look at later. But for now, let's look at how insulin works within the body.

Why insulin makes you fat

Your insulin balance is directly responsible for making your body store food as fat.

Insulin is a hormone produced by the pancreas. Your body releases insulin in response to a rise in blood sugar levels. That's good; it is a vital mechanism that the body could not function without. Too much blood sugar and you would go into a coma; too little and your brain would stop functioning completely. So, the higher the blood sugar, the more insulin is released in an attempt to process the extra sugar. If your body does not use that sugar as energy, it will be stored as body fat. Not just any old body fat, but the fat around your internal organs that creates the spare tyre around your waist; the fat that has far more implications for ill health than any other.

Raised insulin has implications for increased levels of small particle LDL (bad) cholesterol. In fact it is carbohydrate that largely contributes to your dangerous cholesterol levels; not dietary cholesterol as previously thought.

But there's more. Your body, now with a belly full of fat, is producing inflammation that causes your organs to respond less to insulin so it now has to produce more insulin to cope with the incoming sugars. And where does that lead? To more fat storage; a situation known as insulin resistance.

If you struggle with weight gain, cravings and overeating then chances are that you are insulin resistant.

How do I overcome insulin resistance?

The sugar in your body that raises blood sugar comes from dietary carbohydrate. ALL dietary carbohydrates. Some are worse offenders than others, and we do need a certain amount to function effectively. Refined carbohydrates such as white bread, cakes and biscuits are the obvious offenders, but wholemeal bread can raise your blood sugar as much as a slice of stodgy white and other grains and legumes will do so too. Get your insulin response under control and you are halfway to health. How do you do this? By limiting foods with carbohydrate content; namely sugar, grains, legumes and dairy. Vegetables, although sources of carbohydrate, are essential; packed as they are with fibre, life giving vitamins and minerals. They also have little effect upon blood sugar. Fruit is also a valuable source of nutrition but has a greater effect on blood sugar so should be secondary to vegetables; especially to the sedentary individual.

What else affects insulin levels?

The biochemical picture is more complex than just insulin production being affected by carbohydrates, but if one thing will set you free from the stranglehold of empty calories it is getting those blood sugars into balance.

This may seem like a lot to take in and I know it can be overwhelming. This will start to make more and more sense to you as you progress through your Paleo journey and start to be able to identify with the changes that you notice in yourself. This section will be able to give you all the information as to why those changes are happening. Your body really is complex and fascinating and once you understand the changes that are taking place it will all start to make sense and you will feel fantastic.

What other key hormones are involved?

Insulin is only one of the hormones involved in the body's metabolism of food. Hormones are the messengers of the body; set within finely tuned parameters they instruct organs how to act in order to maintain the housekeeping of the human body. When they are thrown off balance everything ends up in chaos; the biological equivalent of an overflowing washing basket and not a clean plate left in the house. The only difference being that an unkempt house is somewhat less likely to cause serious damage to your health. Reversing hormonal dysfunction is fairly simple; not only essential if you are to shed excess weight but a path to wellness, vitality and increased enjoyment of life.

All hormones are made in the body from fatty acids and amino acids. *A diverse and plentiful range of dietary fat and protein* is essential for optimal production of vital molecules within your body.

Glucagon – releases stored sugar

Ingested carbohydrate goes to the liver to be stored as glycogen; the body's store of sugar that ensures we have energy when required. Glucagon, the hormone that manages release of this stored sugar, increases when blood sugar is low and drops when blood sugar is high. Also produced by the pancreas, it works in tandem with insulin; high glucagon means low insulin and reduces appetite. Eating plenty of protein ensures a constant supply of glucagon which in turn leads to decreased appetite and more effective fat burning.

Why carbohydrate is stored as fat

The stores of sugar in the liver are actually fairly low and, as well as capable of keeping itself topped up using fat and protein, the liver needs very little dietary carbohydrate to function effectively. Those with any degree of insulin resistance, especially coupled with a sedentary lifestyle, will need no further glycogen storage and excess dietary carbohydrate will go straight to fat stores instead.

Leptin – manages food intake

Leptin is produced by fat in cells and signals to the brain that food intake (and therefore hunger) needs to be lowered. When your biochemistry is unbalanced the body can become leptin resistant and assume the opposite of full; which, as we are all too aware, means hungry. That leads to more food and, of course, extra insulin. What causes leptin resistance? Extra insulin. Starting to make sense now?

Bring that insulin under control by managing your carbohydrate intake, and your leptin signal can once more be received when it is supposed to.

Ghrelin – another hunger hormone

Ghrelin signals to your brain that the body is no longer hungry, thereby eliminating the desire for more food. Ghrelin levels rise due to lack of sleep, or when you know that a regular mealtime is coming up, and decrease after a meal. Hunger and satiety are not the same thing, but are linked together especially after a meal.

Why you can't stop eating. The next description, of hormones that make you feel full, shows why once you start eating you may find it difficult to stop even though you know you have had enough.

CCK and PYY– make you feel full

Triggered in the small intestine, CCK stimulates digestion of protein and fat as well as playing a role in appetite reduction by increasing the full-feeling known as satiety. Carbohydrates do not trigger CKK as they must be fully digested in order to signal satiety and that happens a lot later in the process of digestion. Therefore by eating protein and fat you will feel fuller after less food, and for longer.

Eating to feel full

PYY, another gut hormone implicated in appetite regulation, is released in the lower section of the small intestine and in the large intestine. PYY signals that the body has had enough food for its requirements and can now stop eating. Eating plenty of insoluble fibre speeds up the passage of food through the digestive tract so that PYY can signal satiety earlier. Baseline PYY levels are thought to be lower in obese individuals.

Cortisol and adrenaline – your stress hormones

Chronic stress is a symptom of modern living that seems to directly correlate with the world's expanding waistline. Chronic symptoms are those that are constantly with us, eating away at our health relentlessly and without respite. Conversely, acute symptoms are those that occur as isolated incidents. The body has evolved finely tuned mechanisms to deal with acute situations, but the unending nature of chronic overload is hugely harmful to health. We discuss stress and how to create a mechanism to control it in Introduction to Yoga and Paleo: 12 Weeks to Change Your Life.

Stress is a double edged sword when it comes to weight gain and obesity. It alters the way in which the body metabolises energy and also encourages us not only to overeat, but to overeat exactly the wrong types of food for our health.

During my career I would continually suffer from stress, it was a daily occurrence and my symptoms really impacted on my everyday life. It was not until I finally left my career that I started to realise just how extreme the instances of stress had become. The first thing I would do when I was stressed would be to reach for some food. It was as though it was the only thing that would calm my mind down and let me forget about the situation for a few minutes. Of course it never stopped at one biscuit. I would easily demolish a whole pack without even noticing in a stress induced frenzy. It was only once I learnt how to control my stress levels that I realised what an impact my previous reactions had on my health and wellbeing.

The two major stress hormones, cortisol and adrenaline, regulate the ways in which our body responds to stressful situations; without them we would not be able to handle stressors of any kind.

Stress hormones cause you to overeat AND store fat

In response to stress, cortisol raises blood pressure and heart rate, increases blood glucose and increases the storage of visceral fat (the harmful fat around your waist); all major physiological factors in metabolic disease.

Adrenaline also takes over when the body is under stress; one of its many roles is to release stored fat for energy. When adrenaline goes up, leptin is decreased; a factor that we now understand leads to overeating.

As with all of the biochemical factors we have looked at, increased exposure leads to resistance, imbalance or dysfunction and the molecules in question cease to do their jobs effectively.

Constant levels of cortisol lead to excessive food intake. Constant levels of adrenaline lead to excessive food intake. Increased resistance to adrenaline diminishes the body's ability to mobilise fat from fat cells to be used for energy. But the importance of stress in relation to weight gain does not end there. Here we look at the concept of reward and show you why when you over-eat it is nearly always something filled with fat and sugar in the same package.

Eating for reward is not just psychological

Saying that you are addicted to food may seem like a blasé joke, but addiction goes far beyond the more obvious choices of alcohol or opiates and could well play a part in your struggle with food intake.

Nothing happens in your body without a reason, and much (if not all) of your behaviour is governed by what is going on inside your body. Yet again, it is that biochemical and hormonal balance that dictates your actions.

The human body is geared for survival; even seemingly abstract responses such as emotions are there to ensure perpetuation of the species. Reward is a biological thing; it keeps us striving for survival by creating the drive to pursue that which is pleasurable. Eating tops the list of functions necessary to our survival so on top of everything else that regulates the process we need to gain pleasure from it too. So enters the subject of palatability. You may enjoy lightly steamed fish with a side of kale, but when confronted with such a thing when you aren't actually physically hungry, or are full, most likely you will turn it down; if that plate contained a large slice of gooey chocolate cake instead then chances are that you would not be able to resist.

The basis of reward in food is that which is palatable, and energy dense; something that often comes in the form of combined fat and sugar. These foods are usually manufactured; or at the very least manufactured in our own kitchen in the form of baking or suchlike. These are the types of food that, although we eat them at other times, we reach for in times of stress or we are unable to refuse in times of stress. We saw before that the stress hormones can lead to compulsive overeating, but what governs the reward system?

It brings us back to leptin and insulin; as most of the roads on this dietary journey do. Leptin should turn off the desire for reward, but in the insulin and leptin resistant body the switch is broken so desire continues; factors that should inhibit the reward sensation of food are effectively removed. Linking directly in to all of the other mechanisms involved in over eating and energy storage, the reward mechanism turns a need for constant food into a need for constant high calorie fat/carb combos. And there is no clear signal that tells the body to STOP.

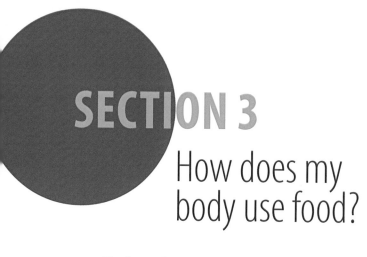

SECTION 3

How does my body use food?

So far we have concentrated on the prime role that insulin plays and looked at the supporting hormonal cast; a subject that focuses largely on carbohydrate. Now let's look at the broader picture of digestion and metabolism. Understanding the physical reasons for eating, and what happens to food once it enters our body, can give us a better insight into why a Paleo approach works and helps to bust open the dietary myths that we have relied on for so long.

What is food?

Food, in the broadest physical sense of the word, is something that we take into our bodies in order to survive; just as we breathe air to provide vital oxygen; without either we would cease to exist.

Broken down into two categories (macronutrients and micronutrients), food serves three main functions essential to life. It provides building blocks, in the form of macronutrients (carbohydrate, protein and fat), and also keeps everything in tip-top condition by utilising micronutrients (vitamins, minerals and other small molecules such as phytochemicals). The third function is that of fuel; food provides us with the means to exist by converting the energy in food to energy that we can use.

In *Paleo: 12 Weeks to Change Your Life* we will explore macronutrients and micronutrients in greater detail; in the context of eating nutrient dense foods.

Which nutrients provide energy?

The short answer to that is all of them. Without sufficient macronutrients and micronutrients we lack the energy required to get through the day. In terms of fuel, it is the macronutrients that provide what we need (backed up very effectively by the micronutrients, as anyone who has suffered from B12 or iron deficiency will soon tell you). But of the three macronutrients the one needed the least is carbohydrate. *That's right; carbohydrate is not your only source of energy, nor is it the most vital.*

How the body uses food for fuel

You may have learnt that the body uses glucose for energy; a fact that is correct but only part of the story. The body converts certain components of food into its own energy currency; a molecule known as ATP. The glucose released from broken down carbohydrate (which remember includes all forms of dietary sugar and starch) is one component used to make ATP. The important thing to take away here is that protein and fats can also be used in the complex pathways that result in ATP production; not just carbohydrate.

Carbohydrates

Carbohydrates are broken down on their journey from the mouth and absorbed, as glucose, into the bloodstream via the small intestine. From here the glucose is taken to the liver, where as we saw earlier it is stored as glycogen with the excess being shunted to the fat cells for storage. As long as you provide your body with a source of dietary carbohydrate it will use it as the primary source of fuel; which means that fat stays where it is.

Fats

Dietary fats and oils are also broken down on their journey through the gastrointestinal tract and eventually arrive at fat cells to be stored as triglycerides. A triglyceride is just a convenient unit of three saturated fatty acids. As well as vital components of many of the body's processes, these fatty acids can be mobilised through the ATP pathway to provide energy. In the absence of dietary carbohydrate, the glycogen stores in the liver will be depleted and the body will use fat as its energy source; a very efficient one at that.

Protein

Protein is the least preferred source of energy for the body but can be converted to ATP if necessary. Proteins are broken down into their component amino acids and sent throughout the body to be used where they are needed. When mobilised for energy production the amino acids are converted to sugars by the removal of nitrogen and then enter the ATP pathway. Protein is essential in the diet for building and repair, as well as playing certain roles in appetite control, but ideally should not be consumed as a primary source of energy.

The message is quite simple; by reducing carbohydrate intake and increasing fat intake you ensure that your body uses fat for fuel, as well as providing the essential fatty acids needed for optimal functioning. Protein intake should be carefully balanced to provide just enough for your body's building and repair needs but not consumed as a primary energy source.

Why increase fat intake?

If carbohydrate intake is to be reduced and protein intake not to exceed requirements then why not just eat less fat too? Won't eating extra fat just replenish my fat stores? The answer to this brings us back to overall calorie intake. As we pointed out at the beginning, the common view that a reduction in overall calories is the only way to lose weight is not entirely correct. Whilst an excess of calories vs expenditure (amongst other factors) will lead to weight gain, there is more to the science of nutrition and weight loss than calories alone.

A body without enough calories is under stress and various feedback mechanisms will kick in that make you hungry, conserve energy and store fat. Calorie restriction or excessive cardio is not a healthy or sustainable route to weight loss; when you stop exercising or start eating the weight will return. Less calories for a sedentary lifestyle is not the answer either; the body needs movement, and plenty of it, for optimum health.

With a reduced carbohydrate intake and an optimum protein ratio of around 20% of total food intake that leaves a calorie deficit that needs to be filled with fat. Not surprisingly, most individuals are fairly fat phobic as we have all been indoctrinated over the years with the low-fat mantra. But if you do not make up your calorie deficit with fat then your weight loss will stall. Your hunger may lead you back to excess carbohydrate intake and back to square one.

I know it is difficult to accept that eating more fat will help you to lose weight. It is an approach that is alien to everyone and goes against all the dieting information we ever thought we knew. There is a common misconception that having a diet higher in fat will mean that you are eating junk food and chocolate for every meal. This is simply not the case. The Paleo diet advocates nutrient dense food which includes fats that are good for you. It is simply not the case that all fats are "bad", you will need to embrace this going forward and judge only once you have seen the results for yourself. You will not only lose weight and look incredible but you will feel full of energy. Trust me – the fat intake in the Paleo diet is necessary for your body to function effectively.

A quick re-cap...

You will need to shed all of the current dietary beliefs that are keeping you from achieving the weight you were designed to be, and embrace a new way of eating that will help you to lose the weight for good:

- The high-carb, low-fat diet that has been prevalent for decades now is clearly not working; obesity rates have risen, not fallen, and modern health is at an all-time low

- Paleo is not a low-carb diet; fruit and vegetables provide the body with all of the dietary carbohydrate it needs

- Your body does not need sugars and starches (dietary carbohydrate), other than those abundant in fruit and vegetables, for energy; even for sports

- It is excess dietary carbohydrate that causes your body to store fat. Dietary fat is essential for optimal health and wellbeing, and can also fuel the body with all of the energy it needs

- Without excess carbohydrate, your body will not only burn off dietary fat very efficiently but is also primed to burn off your excess body fat too

- Paleo is not a high-protein diet; fruit and vegetables actually form the bulk of the diet and protein consumption is just enough to meet your requirements for growth and repair.

The complex biochemistry of this amazing body that we inhabit is exceptionally delicate and needs careful loving maintenance.

A change in diet, one that initially eliminates all possible causes, is the first step to success. That alone will not completely override your unique biochemistry but it should be sufficient to bring insulin and leptin levels to a manageable state. Largely to do with carbohydrate intake, but with other factors inherent in certain foods an issue too, altering your diet to a Paleo framework is about maximising nutrient density and leaving behind the empty and invaluable calorie sources.

As we move on from these intricate details of biochemistry, let's take a broader look at the other ways in which Paleo can improve your health and vitality.

SECTION 4

What are the benefits to adopting a Paleo lifestyle?

So far we have covered your main concern; that of losing weight and keeping it off for good. But the human body is a highly sophisticated system and being overweight has a cascade of ill effects from the way that you feel about yourself to playing host to a number of potentially fatal metabolic diseases.

There is not a single person who would not wish for a healthy body and fully functioning mind within a fit and beautiful body. To be free of illness, or the potential for such, and to have the energy and vitality to be the best that you can be, is for many the elusive Holy Grail. There are some who follow the guidelines to the letter, exercising like Trojans and eating like sparrows, who lead utterly unsatisfying lives in their quest for perceived perfection. There are those who deny the wish to be fit and healthy, squashing their needs beneath an avalanche of fast foods and soft drinks. Then there are the rest of us, who are busy living lives and doing what we can to get through relatively unscathed. Taking care of your body can seem like too much hard work in the face of everything else that needs to be done.

But that is just it. By addressing your biochemical needs and giving your body the nutrient dense foods that it needs and wants, it becomes easy not hard. You begin working with your body not against it. You may imagine that you will spend your days wishing you could eat your weight in cheesecake whilst leaping up and down in the gym. Not so. As your body heals, hunger and cravings slip away. Exercise feels life affirming, not punishment, and almost every area of your physical wellbeing will improve.

With the responsibility for your own health firmly in your own hands and a biochemical balance that you know you can now trust to send you the right signals (and the ability to recognise when it doesn't) you will automatically give your body what it needs, when it needs it. Punishing schedule? Have a high carb day. Feeling particularly hungry? Look at your sleep and eat plenty of protein. Out for coffee with friends? Enjoy it; don't be hard on yourself. A chilled out approach is essential as long as you don't work against your body too much or it will rebel. Rather than the restrictive, even harmful, regime that many people believe Paleo to be, it is actually just a path to understanding your body and devising an individual approach that suits you best. It isn't always easy, and it certainly isn't instant, but the benefits are clear and they will see you through where simply attempting to modify behaviour alone will see you fall at the first craving-shaped hurdle.

Our Paleo plan has been created so that you are in control. It is important that you are able to create a lifestyle that is sustainable for you and not just a passing phase for a few months until you move onto the next dieting approach. I do not believe that following "a diet" for life is sustainable. We are only human and need to incorporate sensible eating decisions into our everyday lives. Our Paleo plan will guide you to a point where you are able to make these sensible decisions and decide what is best for you and your lifestyle. Personally, I decided after my initial Paleo transition that I would start to incorporate some cheese back into my diet. It is my favourite food and life would be miserable without eating it ever again! What I have learnt is how to eat it in moderation and not treat it as a negative action.

Everything within the body is interconnected. Biochemical cascades and pathways work like dominoes and many processes share the same root. Just as the way that we eat and live affect our environment and those around us, all of these factors combine to have a major impact on our health. The imbalances that we already looked at with regards to weight have further implications in our propensity for disease; the key message here is that if you lose the weight, especially the fat around your middle, then you will reverse the markers for many of the major chronic and fatal diseases of our time.

Research indicates that the whole host of degenerative diseases can be linked to the prevalence of industrialised processed food (including seemingly innocent produce) in the modern diet. Refined foods, additives, trans-fats, sugar, unhealthy animals, monoculture cropping and genetic engineering, all play their part. Gluten, especially in modern wheat and other grains, can be shown to have extreme effects on the human body whilst even the gluten-free grains and pulses that rob us of vital nutrients are better left out of our diet.

By taking a holistic approach to your health, and making the necessary changes to your diet and lifestyle, there are a number of improvements that you can expect to see. Although each has separate mechanisms, they all share the same common denominators so eliminating toxins and optimising nutrient intake, as well as following lifestyle changes that are beneficial at the biochemical level, is the most efficient approach; for that reason we highlight only the key benefits below.

Avoid diabetes

Type II diabetes lies at the root of many modern degenerative diseases such as obesity, cancer, heart disease, and neurological disorders. Getting your blood sugar levels in balance and ensuring efficient insulin production is one of the greatest steps you can take towards increased health. On the increase, what used to be termed "adult onset diabetes" is no longer allowed to be called that due to an increased prevalence in children and young people.

Reverse metabolic syndrome

Metabolic syndrome is the term for a group of markers that often occur together and indicate increased likelihood of degenerative disease. They are; abdominal obesity (visceral fat), high blood pressure, elevated blood sugars, high levels of triglycerides in the blood and low levels of HDL (good) cholesterol. Addressing any weight issues and following a diet low in toxins and high in nutrients can significantly decrease or even reverse these markers.

Reduce inflammation

Next to insulin control, one of the most important factors in decreasing the risk of degenerative diseases is reducing inflammation. A natural immune response, inflammation is intended to fight off invaders. And that is exactly what it does. Problem is there are just far too many invaders so that every cell in the body becomes inflamed and even triggers allergic responses; doing all of this means that there is nothing left for fighting off the rest of invading marauders.

Inflammatory conditions such as asthma and joint pain are only the surface manifestations of inflammation; most goes on at the cellular level where you know nothing about it. A healthy immune system is vital against inflammation, but the major culprit is the excess Omega-6 in our bodies that comes from highly processed vegetable oils, practically all processed foods and intensively farmed meat and animal by-products. We discuss Omega-6 further in Paleo: 12 Weeks to Change your Life.

Boost your immune system

A healthy immune system is vital for the body to be the amazing self-healing machine that it is designed to be. Reducing the toxic load (environmental, lifestyle, external and internal) is paramount as well as a daily dose of antioxidant and other life affirming micronutrients. Eliminating gluten is a major factor in reducing inflammation and boosting immunity.

As a teenager I suffered from Chronic Fatigue Syndrome which left me with a weakened immune system and high levels of fatigue for years after I had "recovered". It was perhaps unfortunate that the years which followed my recovery were spent at university embarking on what is probably the worst diet and lifestyle that a person could have! To make matters worse I was a vegetarian and a bad one at that – relying on carbs to get me through every meal. It was not until years later when I embarked on my Paleo journey (having returned to meat eating!) that I realised how what I ate could impact so much on how I felt. For over a decade I had assumed that how I felt was "normal" – learning that this was not the case was life changing for me. I just wish I had known this earlier.

Fatigue? What fatigue

Although fatigue would probably be classed as a symptom rather than an illness, next to weight loss it is probably the number one reason that people choose to follow a Paleo lifestyle. For such a seemingly innocuous thing (what do you mean you're just tired?) fatigue can be just as crippling as any illness, but without a tag to hang to it on and no remedy in sight. Underlying mechanisms of a body in despair will all show themselves as fatigue so the whole system needs attention but an influx of micronutrients on a daily basis will go along way towards making you feel capable of living again. Dealing with any insulin issues and stabilising blood sugar will also stop the nightmare dips that accompany a carbohydrate based diet. Although food remains fuel, it becomes like one of those slow burning fires that never go out rather than a system that constantly requires refuelling; energy literally comes from within.

Feel and look younger

Tired and dehydrated skin, dark rims and bloodshot eyes, excess weight and poor posture do absolutely nothing for your appearance or your sense of wellbeing. With enough healthy fluid (water) and a diet rich in antioxidant, phytochemicals, vitamins and minerals, your skin plumps up, eyes and smile shine, and the excess weight literally melts away. Feeling good makes you look good. Looking good makes you feel even better; we believe it is what they call a self-perpetuating cycle.

Improved mood

Losing weight, looking good and feeling great is enough to make anyone smile, but there are other reasons for your better mood. Mood is largely regulated by your hormonal system and if you have ever burst into tears because you dropped your knife or broken into raucous laughter at a highly inappropriate moment then you know exactly what we mean. With your hormones in balance you can re-join the sane people of the world and feel far more in control. Not only does the influx of nutrients and improved metabolism keep your hormonal levels in check, but eliminating unknowns from your diet and beauty regime can help too; hormone disruptors are absolutely everywhere. Not having to face irritable hunger every few hours goes a long way too.

Appropriate stress responses

We all cope in different ways so when we say "appropriate" we mean "appropriate to you". A body that is constantly flooded with stress hormones is the quickest path to ill health, but as we cannot remove most stressors we need to alter how we deal with them. Regulation of insulin and other hormones clears the way to seeing things in perspective, whilst a physically fit and healthy body is better equipped to deal with life in general. After that, techniques in stress management, regular relaxation, and putting a little more time into your own self development will help to create excellent coping strategies for whatever life throws at you. This is explored in depth in Paleo: 12 Weeks to Change Your Life and Introduction to Yoga.

Improved and restorative sleep

The power of good quality sleep has become a huge issue right now, with research, techniques and discussions at the forefront of practically every health movement. Poor quality sleep has the power to affect the functioning of your body in a myriad of ways; increased hunger and fat storage, hormonal disruption, chronic inflammation, oxidative stress, aging, memory loss and depression. By learning to tune in to your body's needs and set everything back into sync you will learn to deal with stress and restore yourself with quality sleep every night.

A healthy heart

The entire mainstream view of a healthy diet is based on outdated ideas from half a century ago concerned with keeping a heart healthy; namely that dietary cholesterol and saturated fat are responsible for heart disease. This has plausible links to the catastrophic picture of ill health, obesity, diabetes and heart disease that we see before us today, borne out by a low-fat, high-carb diet full of processed, often "healthy", foods full of highly processed vegetable oils.

The majority of risk factors presented for heart disease can be prevented or reversed by dietary and lifestyle changes. As well as a diet devoid of the horrors described above, a good intake of heart healthy nutrients, including Omega-3 fats from oily fish and monounsaturated fats from olive oil, avocado and some nuts, should help keep your heart healthy. On top of that you need to move more, sleep well and address any stress management issues that you may have.

Improved digestion

The health of your digestive system does not necessarily manifest as digestive issues, although it can lead to problems with itching, wind, bloating, irregular stools and even abdominal pain. Up there with restoring insulin balance and reducing inflammation, addressing the overall health of your gut is a vital step along the path to health. A gut imbalance can manifest as depression, psoriasis or even heart disease. There are two factors involved in the health of your gut; bacterial levels (gut flora) and the integrity of the intestinal lining: problems in one often indicate issues with the other.

Your entire intestinal tract is home to millions of bacteria, mostly beneficial to health in some way or another, but eating a diet high in sugar, processed foods, refined carbs and dietary toxins such as gluten, can upset the delicate balance and cause the less than favourable bacteria to crowd out the beneficial strains. Taking medication, especially antibiotics, and chronic stress also contribute.

Inflammation and irritation of the gut lining can lead to increased permeability that lets large protein molecules and other unwanted substances pass through into the bloodstream. The body then recognises these particles as the intruders that they are and mounts an immune response. Health of the intestinal lining is essential to the health of your immune system.

In order to rebuild healthy gut flora and restore the delicate lining of the tract you need to learn to manage stress and avoid all sources of food toxins. Eating sweet potato (a fermentable fibre) is said to be good for restoration of the lining. Otherwise a good quality pro-biotic supplement should help.

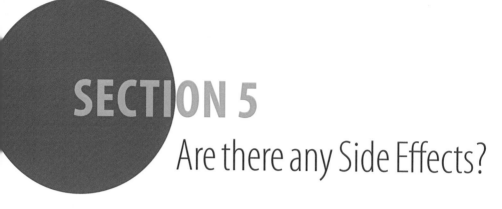

SECTION 5

Are there any Side Effects?

One aspect of starting a Paleo diet that many guides do not mention is the possibility of side effects. Painting a picture of immediate glowing health may be very good for sales and the reputation of the movement as a whole but if you get caught short feeling less than healthy it can be bewildering and disheartening; especially when you are expecting impending miracles.

If you embarked on a detox program, often seen as a beauty regime or spa type of treatment, you would be advised to clear the whole weekend, make the place all floaty and feminine (with the odd scented candle or two), and basically prepare for the worst. When you embark on Paleo, which is far more detoxing than a day long juice fast, no-one seems to take this side of it into account.

Chances are that you will start the plan and immediately feel the benefits; most people do exactly that and never look back. There is no particular rhyme or reason to those who may feel worse than others, but if you come from a place of completely empty nutrition, high sugar and refined carb intake, or high caffeine intake, then you may experience anything from a slight headache to full blown flu-like symptoms.

I have to say that I did not experience any negative side effects when I started the Paleo diet. I was actually surprised at how quickly my body adapted and how great I felt within a matter of days. If you do feel any side effects then please do not let this put you off – it will pass and you will start to feel the benefits so stick with it.

Your favourite foods may be the very ones that harm you; when symptoms are masked you could have been carrying various food intolerances around with you without even realising it. Often it can be those foods that we eat a lot of that catch us in a contradictory cycle of addiction and intolerance. If you eat a lot of bread, for example, then you may find that you have a full blown reaction to it being removed from your diet. Going from high caffeine to no caffeine is bound to give you a headache and if you have previously eaten a lot of highly processed foods those toxins are going to start fleeing your body like rats from a ship.

You could come from a place of fairly balanced nutrition, according to the mainstream view. Whilst more likely to lead to a smoother ride, this is no indication that you aren't harbouring issues with wheat or dairy that can cause initial havoc when no longer consumed. What we will say however is that if you have a rough time of detoxing then it really shows you how much harm your diet has been doing to your body. When, later down the line, you experiment with re-introducing certain foods you may experience symptoms that reveal the extent of your intolerance and decide that staying with a completely clean diet is the way forward for you.

These early days are when you really learn to listen to your body. The effects of an influx of vitamins, minerals and phytochemicals (especially if you are seriously deficient) will be felt virtually immediately; even if they are underlying the symptoms of detox you can feel them pushing through like a sense of vitality under your skin.

You will be thirsty; drink LOTS of water to help flush out toxins. Don't overdo it though; listen to your body.

You may wake up feeling ravenous, or you may barely have the energy for food. Some of the foods on the plan are very restorative and light whilst others are going to give you a dose of red meat protein exactly when you are most likely to need it. Everyone is different, but hopefully these foods are well timed to suit your utmost needs.

You may have no energy; don't push it. Sometimes, gentle stretching or getting up and moving around helps. If it doesn't, then rest; suitable exercise is built into the 7 day plan, but judge your own limits. If you are feeling energetic then get started on your exercise programme by reading Tabata Transformation or if you want to take things a bit slower try Introduction to Yoga. Again, this is about listening to your body's needs. You know from the previous chapters about biochemistry and behaviour so you have a clue about what to listen for. Craving a bread bun? That's not real. Thirsty? That's real. Tired? Investigate further; you may need to move or you may need to rest. Ask your body and trust your judgement; unless it asks for ice cream.

Headache? If you need analgesia to get through it then do it. Flu symptoms? Take time off and go to bed. This time right now has to take precedence; you need to do this. Cold turkey from forbidden foods is essential whilst you detox, but there are certain food strategies built into our 7 day plan to help you give your body what you may need.

The 7 day plan is quite energy-dense. Everything is nutrient-dense too so it's fine, but at this stage you may need more calories than you do later down the line. It needs to be low-carb at this stage; it won't be that way forever. Low-carb can make you feel restless at night so we have included sweet potatoes and bananas to combat this; magnesium rich foods may also help so we have included plenty of those too.

The protein, fat and carbohydrate balance is perfectly tuned to weight loss and the ingredients have been chosen for maximum influx of vitamins. It is actually unlikely that you will feel any cravings; if you do, it won't be for something that your body actually needs. If you do need to snack, then snack on berries, fruit and nuts. Keep a bar of dark chocolate in the drawer and have a few squares if you need to. Eventually, in fact by the time you reach the end of your first couple of weeks, you probably won't want that snack.

When I first started the Paleo transition I found it useful to eat snacks on a daily basis. It helped to keep me in a routine and it was something I would focus on for a break at work. I found that natural fruit bars were a real treat and very satisfying. I would stock up on "nakd" bars (available in health food shops) and have them with a cup of green tea. I found that they satisfied any urge for something sweet and they felt like a real treat. I still look forward to them now. Having some mixed nuts and berries is also a really lovely treat. You will soon find that the snacks you usually crave are actually not as nice as you remembered and that any sugar craving can easily be filled guilt free. So much of snacking is psychological so try to really think about why you want that snack; I would freely admit my snacks are often as a distraction to my work or an excuse to take a break. There is nothing wrong with this; just so long as they don't happen every 10 minutes!

If it is hard, you will get through this sooner than you think. If it isn't; then great. You may find that the transition is easy and doesn't really affect you too much or you may find that your entire life changes during the 7 day plan; as over the top as it may sound, food is a powerful thing and really is capable of effecting monumental change. Or you might decide that it really isn't for you. Do try though; give it a chance through the good or the bad and then make an informed decision as to whether it is for you. We would recommend that you try to complete the 12 week programme as set out in Paleo: 12 Weeks to Change Your Life before you make any decisions as to what foods you may wish to re-introduce into your diet. Now, finally, we get to look at food.

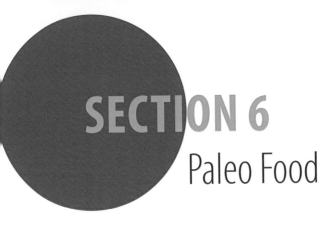

SECTION 6
Paleo Food

Below is the lowdown on the foods relevant to Paleo eating. At the back of the book you will find a colour coded list; by no means comprehensive, but it will nonetheless provide inspiration and a head start and assist with making good food decisions when out and about.

Which foods does the Paleo diet eliminate?

Grains

Found in grains are three substances considered detrimental to human health; gluten, lectins, and phytic acid. Gluten is one of many proteins in wheat and other grains that can damage the body. Not limited to the symptoms of celiac disease, or even those of a noticeable intolerance, the ravaging effects of gluten can have ill effects on everyone.

Lectins, also present in grains, cause the body to mount an immune attack against its own healthy cells; a situation that can lead to auto immune diseases. Phytic acid binds to certain essential minerals and carries them out of the body, leading the way for mineral imbalances; it is known as an anti-nutrient.

For these reasons, grains and cereals such as barley, buckwheat, corn, oats, rice, wheat, and spelt are not permitted in the Paleo diet. This includes all of their derivatives such as flours, and all goods made from these flours. These grains and cereals can find their way into everything in the form of fillers, flavourings and additives; even in products labelled as whole or health foods.

Grains, especially when ground into flour, form the basis of carbohydrate in the diet. Bread, pasta, noodles, rice, couscous and others all contribute, whether wholegrain or not, to the excessive carbohydrate load on the body and, alongside refined sugars are the biggest reason for insulin resistance in individuals. They also help to provide the greatest number of empty calories. See grains; think sugar.

Legumes

Legumes also contain lectins and phytic acids so are eliminated from the Paleo diet. Thought of as protein foods, beans and pulses are actually three quarters carbohydrate so have noticeable effects upon blood sugar levels and insulin response.

This includes all of the pulses and beans, including lentils, black eyed peas, chickpeas, and red beans. Also included here are soy beans in all forms, and peanuts (which are not actually a nut). Green peas and beans that are eaten as vegetables are however fine to eat.

Dairy

Homogenised, pasteurised dairy produce from industrially farmed animals is a veritable catalogue of dietary misdemeanours. Fat molecules are disrupted, enzymes are destroyed and the poor diet and health of the animal leaves little room for nutrients in her milk. High levels of oestrogen in milk can contribute to hormonal imbalance. Milk sugar (lactose) and protein (casein) was never designed to be ingested by the human body and can cause intolerance symptoms in many people; many of them not recognisable until eliminated and re-introduced in isolation. If you decide to re-introduce dairy then choose unpasteurised raw produce from grass-fed animals. There are health benefits and certainly flavour benefits associated with certain high quality dairy products.

Refined sugar

As far as your body is concerned, sugar is sugar. Even dietary starch is sugar to your bloodstream and hormonal processes. Some sugars are digested so quickly that they cause an immediate spike in blood sugar followed by the less immediate crash accompanied by irritability, fatigue and possibly even a headache. Others are metabolised less quickly but will still end up as stored fat. Some sources of sugar have absolutely no nutrient value whatsoever whilst others come with vitamins, minerals, fibre and phytonutrients; such as fruit.

An ancient natural sweetener, honey, may come with plenty of health benefits but will have the same overall effect as table sugar so should be used in moderation. Agave syrup, touted as a health food, is really bad stuff on a par with high fructose corn syrup; avoid it. Hidden sugars are everywhere from on the outside, and even the inside, of your supermarket free range ham to "healthy" wholegrain cereal products. Be very wary of any food that comes pre-packed and by law needs an ingredient label; if you need to read a label then you are already one step removed from the ideal diet.

Take your sugar, and perfectly natural desire for sweet food, minimally and in the form of fresh fruit. You may be surprised how little you actually miss sugar. If you do want a treat then you can use raw honey or organic maple syrup as a natural sweetner when making Paleo treats. But remember they should only be consumed as a treat and in moderation.

Vegetable oils

Modern vegetable oils are highly processed (the only way to squeeze oil from a hard seed or grain) and easily oxidised by heat or light. This means that in the body they form free radicals and unstable molecules that lead to inflammatory conditions and general chaos. Highly processed vegetable oils, and their chemically mutated offspring trans-fats, are the reason for the imbalance of Omega-6 to Omega-3 in the population at large.

Don't use cheap, or otherwise, cooking oils; vegetable oil, corn oil, sunflower oil all come under this heading. Also avoid processed foods containing these things; practically everything does from your expensive "deli-style" olives to ice cream. Choose cold pressed nut oils, olive oil and animal fats.

Additives

It goes without saying that additives in food should be banned from your diet. Again, as ingredients that you wouldn't consider cooking with, they find their way into anything that requires a label. Stick to fresh produce and prepare your food from scratch.

Soft drinks and fruit juices

You should avoid drinking anything cold that isn't water. Not only will you avoid nasties and sugar but you will have the glow of a supermodel. That said, green juices and some enriched smoothies made at home can provide extra nutrients and we provide some tasty recipes for juices and smoothies in Paleo: 12 Weeks to Change Your Life.

If you do want to drink some fruit juice try to make a fresh juice yourself, you can buy juicers very cheaply and you can be as inventive as you like with juice combinations. If this is not an option then make sure that any shop bought juice is not from concentrate.

Refined salt

Refined salt contains additives that make it flow. Choose sea salt for better flavour and mineral content; flaked sea salt is easy to control with your fingertips rather than a grinder. Keep salt within minimum safe levels and ensure you get enough fluids. You may need to experiment with the levels that suit your body.

Which foods can you eat freely?

Vegetables

Vegetables form the bulk of any healthy diet; nutrient dense but low in calorie, they are packed full of fibre, vitamins, minerals and phytochemicals. The composition of every plant is different from the next with each containing hundreds of different minerals and phytochemicals. The beneficial effect of these natural substances on human and animal health cannot be repeated too many times or replicated in a laboratory. Eat as wide a range of fresh produce as you can as these nutrients work synergistically; that is to say that their sum is greater than their parts. Choosing vegetables based on colour by filling your basket with as many colours as are possible is the best way to ensure the greatest range. On a Paleo diet you will have had your 5 a day by lunchtime and it is this part of your diet that will provide you with all the vitality you need to face life full on.

Herbs

Fresh herbs, whether straight from the garden or out of a packet, are full of the same goodness as fruit and vegetables and bring life to your cooking. Get used to throwing huge handfuls of parsley or mint in salads and bunches of thyme in the slow cooker. As well as adding flavour and vibrancy to your food, experiment with different types of herbs for their therapeutic value; teas and tisanes, beauty products and even cleaning products. Having herbs always to hand will make a big difference to your food.

Fruit

Fruits contain different yet more variations on the vital nutrients theme and are therefore an essential part of the mix. They are however full of sugar too so elicit the same responses as table sugar. Some fruits have less impact on the glycaemic load and you should choose these varieties; berries are the best and their bright colours bring a boost of phytochemicals, apples and pears are full of soluble fibre, and citrus fruits are packed with vitamins.

Bananas get a bad press because of their sugar load but they are great for desserts or if you feel in need of a carbohydrate boost. Try to keep your fruit intake limited especially if you are not very active. However, if you are carrying out regular exercise then you will be able to burn off the excess sugar much more easily. You may find that you eat more fruit to start with than you feel the need for further down the line.

Meat

Contrary to popular belief, meat does not form the basis of Paleo eating. Yes it is considered vital to human health and is likely to be present at each meal but excessive slabs of steak are not the story here.

Let's begin with a statement; meat is not the enemy. There are various reasons for the common belief that meat is either unnecessary or should be limited. The most compelling, for most people, is the issue of saturated fat and cholesterol. Saturated fat, apart from some plant oils such as coconut and palm, is the fat of animals. Even 30 years ago most people fried their eggs in lard and cooked their chips in dripping; not because it was trendy but because it was the accepted way of doing things.

Then the low-fat, high-carb recommendations came along and turned the whole thing on its head. More recently the perceived horrors of saturated fat are being discredited one by one but it will be a long time before the stigma has faded and the powers that be raise their hands in defeat. It has long been conceded that dietary cholesterol has nothing to do with the total amount of cholesterol in your body. Put this together with the fact that most animal (saturated) fats are a roughly balanced mix of saturated fatty acids and monounsaturated fatty acids and the shoddily built case against animal fat begins to collapse.

The other theme is environmental and the view that too much meat is bad for the planet. Too much industrial meat is disastrous for the planet. The animals that it raises are unhealthy and produce substandard cheap meat. These same animals are fed cheap grain that has taken over vast tracts of our planet and is slowly strangling our environment. Those fats we were talking about? Grain, as it does humans, makes animals fat. Not good fat but Omega-6 laden fat; just like us. Flabby, greasy meat from undernourished animals is doing no one any good; in fact it harms the animals, the environment and the people it feeds. Let's not even further muddy the waters with talk of pesticides, antibiotics and everything else that has to support a failing monoculture; just be aware that these things are there in the industrial meat supply.

On the other hand, grass-fed animals live under much improved conditions and enjoy a diet full of lush grass and the other varied flora that should flourish in a traditional mixed farm setting. The goodness of their diet translates into the quality of their meat. Ridding the world of industrial meat fed by industrial grain would result in a far more sustainable meat supply and more nutritious meat.

What about quantity? A lot of industrially processed meat ends up in burgers, chicken nuggets, substandard cooked meats and salamis. A more traditional approach to meat preparation and cookery would automatically eliminate the need for all of these products and make better use of the animal. In a hypothetical diet of 2000 calories, with a protein content of under 30%, that's 600 calories from meat (don't forget fish) or the equivalent of less than 300g of steak. Considering the average portion of meat or hamburger is 250g then that suddenly doesn't seem so excessive after all does it?

Humans need protein, in the form of essential amino acids to survive. Meat contains all of these essential amino acids, along with a healthy dose of essential fatty acids, vitamins and minerals. Protein also elicits satiety responses and takes longer to digest, making it the ideal slow burning food. Eating meat quite simply gives you a lot of nutritional bang for your buck. Choose a wide range of meat, paying attention to parts of the animal that you may never have considered before. Grass-fed, free-range meat is the best choice of all.

Fish and shellfish

Fish also provides a good source of animal protein. Oily fish are excellent sources of Omega-3 fatty acids; the canned varieties with bones also provide calcium and the vitamin D needed for the body to utilise it. Choose fish in season, from reputable suppliers and don't be afraid to try new varieties. Shellfish are also a cheap source of animal protein and come with a healthy dose of essential minerals.

Eggs

Eggs are the most inexpensive form of protein available and are one of the most complete sources of food available to us; it goes without saying to choose fresh free-range eggs. Don't limit yourself to hens egg's; look for quail, duck and interesting variations.

Nuts and seeds

Nuts and seeds should be eaten in moderation as they are hugely energy dense. A good source of protein, healthy fats, and minerals, nuts and seeds also contain lectins and phytic acid so are best sprouted; that said a handful of raw nuts or seeds adds variety and texture to your meals and make a handy snack.

Fats

Fats are essential for our health and vital in the kitchen for preparing delicious food. Light olive oil and animal fats such as dripping, lard or goose fat are best for cooking as they oxidise less easily than other fats. Keep extra virgin olive oil for salads and dressings, as well as cold-pressed nut oils. Coconut oil is the Paleo cooking oil of choice but its robust flavour does not suit all foods; match your fat to the food you are cooking. Food is as much about flavour as it is about health.

Condiments, seasonings, and shelf food

Most ready-made condiments have long lists of ingredients that include vegetable oil, forms of sugar and additives. If you do need to use something from a bottle, make sure it is unadulterated. Spice blends and ground spices in packets are often full of fillers and preservatives; grinding your own spices is the best way to go. Good quality chilled chicken stock can be useful; although homemade is preferable. As long as food is additive free, and made from Paleo ingredients, you can take all the short cuts that you need.

What can you eat and drink occasionally?

The foods listed below are acceptable in moderation; not necessarily bad for you, and even with health benefits, they are also sources of sugar that need to be kept to a minimum.

- Fruit juice

- Alcohol

- Dark chocolate

- Dried fruit

- Raw honey

Feel free to drink unsweetened herbal teas and allow yourself one cup of caffeinated tea or coffee each day, either black or with coconut milk or almond milk, if you feel that life would be miserable without it.

A detailed discussion on Paleo food is continued in Paleo: 12 Weeks to Change Your Life which examines closely why Paleo eliminates certain foods in order to optimise health and weight loss.

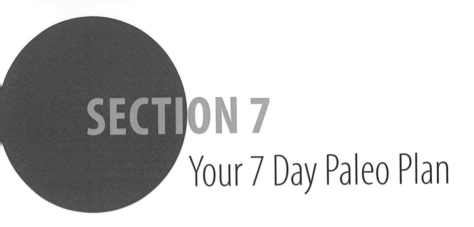

SECTION 7
Your 7 Day Paleo Plan

Introduction to Paleo has been designed to address every need of those making the transition to a Paleo lifestyle. We have provided 7 daily worksheets that contain a breakdown of the meals for the day and notes on any advance preparation required.

Our Paleo plan has been designed to help you transform every aspect of your health and wellbeing to achieve a sustainable and healthy lifestyle. This goes much further than just changing your diet. We believe that exercise is an important part of your transformation. Not only will it greatly assist with weight loss and toning, it will provide a feeling of self-confidence and self-belief that will change your whole outlook on life. We therefore recommend that you incorporate *Tabata Transformation* and/or *Introduction to Yoga* into your Paleo journey.

During your initial 7 day transition we have included exercise tips on each daily worksheet. We have accounted for the fact that you may be feeling some side effects so the exercise suggestions are based upon gentle exercise and movement that will enable your body to adjust to the change in diet. If you feel able, then please start incorporating more intensive exercise such as the *Tabata Transformation* programme into your routine during the 7 day plan.

We suggest that you begin the plan at the start of the working week, or even take some time out whilst you concentrate on getting the best start with Paleo that you can. Before beginning you will need to do a complete shop and also look at some of the advance preparation required to make the transition to Paleo eating as smooth as possible.

The daily plan has been designed in such a way that the nutritional elements meet your overall requirements as well as addressing the specific needs of the early days of a new way of eating. You can then mix and match the recipes going forward with your Paleo journey.

We believe in good food as well as good nutrition and living. To this end the recipes have all been created by a chef with a view to increasing your competence in the kitchen and understanding that flavour is everything when it comes to food. If you want to change, amend or add to any of the recipes then please do so. We would encourage you to actively experiment with flavours to see what works best for you.

Throughout the plan you will find inspiration on approaching your life in ways that improve your wellbeing and therefore fuel your weight loss. Using the very latest research from the fields of life coaching and self-management, these tips will encourage mindfulness and make sure you keep on top of all the facets of a Paleo lifestyle that will result in optimal health and vitality.

The eventual goal of your Paleo journey is to be self-aware and self-managed. This takes a little effort, but to have a diet and lifestyle that fits you and only you is well worth it. Once you complete your transitional phase (which we recommend is after completing Paleo: 12 Weeks to Change Your Life) you can look ahead to re-introducing certain foods one by one, fine-tuning your individual body needs, and taking a more flexible approach. In order to do this, you need to learn the skills of being both self-aware and self-managed.

Measuring your progress

In order to accurately track your progress we would recommend that you take a full set of body measurements at the beginning of the programme, along with photographs. Try to concentrate not only on the lumps and bumps, but your overall look of wellbeing. This can be a really helpful tool to accurately assess your progress.

You will also know within yourself how you are progressing. You will see a difference when you look in the mirror and will notice how your clothes are fitting. You should also notice how soft your skin begins to feel and how much brighter your complexion; feel the spring in your step and the tension leave your shoulders. These factors can be a great indicator as to your progress and also fantastic motivation.

You may also want to weigh yourself but try not to get hung up on it, but all self-development needs a record in order to continually assess progress. We assess how to accurately measure your weight loss and set appropriate goals in Tabata Transformation. We would recommend that you review this before you start.

What measurements do I need to take?

We have set out below the body measurements that we recommend you take before starting the programme. If you would like to take additional measurements then please do so.

Measuring Tips: Make sure that you stand tall and straight and breathe normally – if you breathe in you are only cheating yourself! Always make sure that the tape measure is level around your body and that it is parallel to the floor. The tape measure should be close to your skin but should not be constraining. To get the most accurate measurements you will need someone to assist you.

BODY AREA	MEASUREMENT
CHEST	Stand with your arms stretched out to the side and measure around the area just under your bust/pecs
BUST	Stand with your arms stretched out to the side and measure around the fullest part of your bust
WAIST	Measure around your "natural" waist which is the narrowest part of your upper body
LOWER WAIST	Measure around the widest part of your waist. This is usually at the belly button
HIP	Find your hip bone and measure around this area
BOTTOM	Measure around the fullest part of your bottom/hip area
BICEPS	Stand with your arm out to the side and measure around the fullest part of your upper arm.
THIGHS	Stand with one leg forward and measure around the fullest part of your thigh
CALF	Measure around the widest part of your calf

How often should I check my progress?

At the beginning of the programme you should decide how often you will have a "weigh in" to check on your progress. We would recommend that these are kept at least two weeks apart. You should take a note of your weight, measurements and any other observations and take updated photographs wearing the same clothing. Please avoid the temptation to weigh yourself every day; your body naturally goes through fluctuations on a daily basis and this can be easily mistaken for weight gain.

We wish you every success on your weight loss journey; keep the information that you have learnt throughout Introduction to Paleo at the forefront of your mind and enjoy these first steps towards sustained weight loss. Learn to listen to your body and relax your mind. Enjoy the new flavours and textures you will discover and have fun preparing food that will nourish you; body and mind.

Are you ready? Let's go.

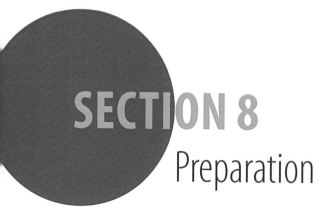

SECTION 8
Preparation

When it comes to making time for self-supporting practices such as healthy eating and exercise, a little planning goes a very long way. In fact, learning to plan effectively is one of the key actions in any successful lifestyle; it is when you are unprepared that you become most likely to drop the ball.

Read the plan

We suggest reading through the whole plan, including the recipes, to familiarise yourself with the tasks ahead. Does the meal structure fit in with your life? This way of eating may be completely new to you and present you with time management challenges along the way but are there any particular non-negotiable obstacles like early morning or late evening meetings coming up? If so, then you may want to think about using available time for advance preparation or swapping out some of the meals to suit your timetable.

I found that my main downfall when it came to food was just not being prepared. I would often have long days at work and would use every minute I had outside of work to catch up with friends or sleep. I found that by planning what I was going to eat a couple of days at a time I was able to prepare in advance which made it very easy for me to stick to the eating plan. It really didn't take as much time as I thought it would and made such a difference to my outlook and determination to succeed. It also helped me to save a lot of money which would otherwise have been spent on last minute convenience food – I was shocked at how much the weekly savings added up to – all as a result of a bit of preparation and some tupperware boxes!

Advance preparation

Eating a cooked breakfast can be a challenge (in fact for some eating breakfast at all is a new concept) that may require a little forethought. Breakfast on Monday for instance involves peppers and mushrooms; you may wish to chop these ready the night before; cooking an omelette first thing may seem taxing, but it really does take minutes and you will feel the benefits right up to lunchtime. We have included kitchen planning tips in your daily meal planner where relevant.

Flexibility

We appreciate that everyone leads very hectic and busy lives and that sometimes it is just not possible to plan ahead as much as we would like and sometimes we just have days where we simply can't be bothered. This is completely normal! Whilst we have provided you with bespoke meal plans and recipes you may sometimes prefer to prepare a quick and simple meal that doesn't need instructions. This is perfectly fine. Whilst we would recommend that you try to follow the meal plan we have provided as often as you can, as this has taken all your nutritional requirements into account, we appreciate that sometimes you just want something else. Whether this is just a steak and some steamed vegetables to a simple vegetable soup everyone has their own "go to" meals that they can rely on when needed.

My quick and easy meal was steak and vegetables. If I had a really long day at work I would be able to get in and put the steak on and this would then be nearly cooked by the time I got changed. While the steak was resting I would put the vegetables on (I would love to include green leafy vegetables with steak) and within 15 minutes of walking in the door I could be in my pj's having a really tasty meal that I loved. If I had the energy I would also poach an egg. Just divine!

Organise your space

Start in a clean, clutter free environment. Organising your kitchen space so it is a pleasure to be in and making sure that an endless trail of laundry and tidying up does not derail you is a relevant concern. We are not suggesting that you reorganise all the cupboards or decorate your home but a clean and tidy space can work wonders for a stress free mind. Clearing the clutter from the bedroom to create a calming restorative space is an absolute must. We have included tips on optimising your sleep environment throughout the 7 day plan.

Shop ahead for the week

Doing the shopping all in one go frees up time during the week and can also prevent any un-necessary purchases. Use our shopping list at the end of the book to make life easier and enjoy a fridge full of vibrant natural produce; nothing spurs on unhealthy eating choices like an empty fridge. There will also be weekly shopping lists provided in *Paleo: 12 Weeks To Change Your Life.*

Keep a diary

Keeping a journal may seem like just another way to eat into your available time but it can be a powerful tool for change and may save you time in the long run. There are no quick fixes in life and successful, sustainable change involves a lot of hard work. Do the leg work now though and you will congratulate yourself further down the line on a job well done.

We will remind you throughout the weekly planner of the importance of a holistic approach that addresses far more than the food you eat, as well as tips on getting the most from your endeavours. This will ease you into the practice of using reflection to keep yourself moving towards your goals, but we suggest keeping a journal for as long as you need to; one dedicated workbook is a good way to achieve this and setting aside time at the beginning or the end of the day is recommended. It may also be prudent to jot down thoughts or actions as they occur.

Practice stress management and self-awareness

Writing down your thoughts and actions, reflecting on what you have written and incorporating that information into your plans is the key to any self-improvement program. In Paleo: 12 Weeks To Change Your Life we cover these skills in detail, with a focus on stress management and self-awareness.

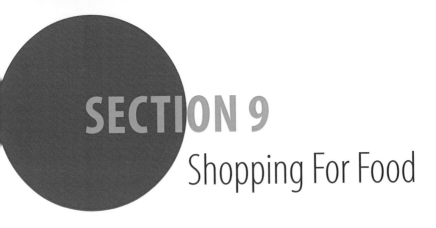

SECTION 9
Shopping For Food

Depending on your usual shopping, cooking, and eating habits, buying the food for your Paleo lifestyle may be no different to before or represent a huge change. Modern shopping issues are rife with argument about what is right and what is wrong and can be confusing to say the very least. We do not want to make this week any more of an upheaval than it has to be but food security is very much a concern of the Paleo movement and as such deserves a mention here.

How do I know what to buy?

Any search on the Paleo diet will show you that the recommended shopping list involves free-range grass-fed local meat, local organic vegetables and a whole host of items that can be beyond the budget of many households. Depending on your current diet, shifting to a whole foods approach can seem expensive but it does even out and can even save you money. We have become so used to cheap industrial food that the real thing has lost all of its value; we are probably prepared to spend more on any other portion of the household expenses than we are on food and in a budgeting setback food is often the first thing to feel the cuts. *Paleo: 12 Weeks to Change Your Life* explores these food issues in further detail but here are some pointers to help you make the all-important decisions.

Choose local produce above organic. It will be in season and therefore have more flavour, more nutrients and a reasonable price tag. Local food is often grown with more natural principles and although it doesn't carry the costly organic certification it could be virtually organic anyway. An added benefit to buying local is that you can build a rapport with an actual person as oppose to self-serve environment in a faceless corporation. When shopping in a large supermarket these days, quite often the only people you come into contact with are the ever-present shelf stackers.

Where budget allows, choose supermarket organic above supermarket non-organic. Mass produced organic food pretty much makes a mockery of the movement by barely slipping through the required certification and then shipped half way around the world; look at where it comes from and make a decision from there. At least with supermarket organic you are still guaranteed some protection from pesticides and the havoc caused by industrial farming.

A diet of mainly meat and vegetables at least cuts out many shopping decisions automatically. Go for the best quality and most sustainable sources that you can afford; you will become familiar with your particular shopping environment and adept at seeing the links between appearance with quality and flavour. At the end of the day, a diet of the cheapest produce is still going to be far better for your health than a diet of processed industrial food. If it needs an ingredients label then chances are you can manage without it.

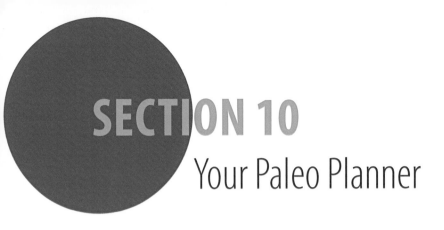

SECTION 10
Your Paleo Planner

Day 1 of your Paleo Journey

Welcome to the first day of your weight-loss journey; we think congratulations are in order for taking back control of your health and your life. At this stage you are most likely to feel excited about the changes ahead, maybe a little wary of feeling hungry, and perhaps concerned about the time you will need to create meals. You are unlikely to feel any physical changes at this stage so take the time to concentrate on enjoying your time in the kitchen and savouring the food on your plate. Drink plenty of water and if you feel the need to snack, reach for fruit in the form of apples, pears and berries or a handful of nuts.

Enjoy your meals -

BREAKFAST - Spinach, Pepper and Mushroom Omelette
LUNCH - Mackerel Salad Nicoise
DINNER - Lemon and Sage Roast Chicken; Root Mash with Paprika and
           Fennel Seed
DESSERT - Banana, Coconut and Almond Ice Cream

Nutrition - Fibre 100%+, Sodium 100%+, Potassium 100%+, Iron 100%+, Magnesium 100%+, Vitamin A 100%+, Vitamin K 18%, Vitamin B12 100%+, Vitamin B6 100%+, Vitamin C 19%, Vitamin D 1%, Vitamin E 100%+

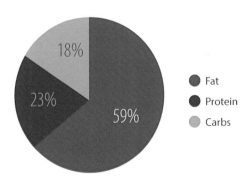

Exercise

This week represents some fairly intense changes into the way you eat and plenty of food for thought too. Exercise is also an integral part of a Paleo lifestyle and essential to your weight loss goals but for this week let's concentrate on simply introducing more movement into your life. The Paleo principles of fitness are the opposite of harmful intense cardio or over reliance on machines, focusing rather on functional strength and flexibility training, with short bursts of intense activity.

This is why Tabata and Yoga work incredibly well alongside Paleo to help you reach your fitness and weight loss goals; both are covered in detail in *Tabata Transformation* and *Introduction to Yoga*. As well as exploring these disciplines, and dependent upon your energy levels, spend this week practising ways to increase your daily movement levels. Start today by focusing on moving with energy; whether you are doing housework, walking up stairs or popping to the shop, do it with determination and act like you mean it!

Stress Management

Take some time today to consider the sources of stress in your life. Do you suffer from a constant bombardment of daily issues or are you coping with particular circumstances? Write down in your journal, all the sources of stress in your life. We would recommend that you review *Paleo: 12 Weeks to Change Your Life* and *Introduction to Yoga* to consider the impact of stress in more detail and the importance of adopting a mechanism to help you cope with stress.

Sleep

As we have seen, quality of sleep has a major impact upon every area of your life and consequently your health and weight loss goals. Take some time to think about your current sleep patterns and how they affect your daily life. Make a record each day of how well you slept the night before.

Self-Awareness

Self-awareness is the key to getting the most out of your life and sadly the piece of the puzzle that often needs the most attention. Self-awareness comes through constant reflection and is a lifelong process of development and growth. Often dismissed by those who would possibly benefit the most there is plenty to learn by exploring your place in the world and you only need take it as far as you feel comfortable. Begin today by considering how well you actually understand yourself and record your thoughts.

Planning

What practical steps can you take today that will make life easier tomorrow? After dinner, strip the remaining meat from the chicken carcasses and make Chicken Stock with the bones.

You could get ahead for tomorrow by preparing the Chicken Salad with Olives and Artichokes for lunch, the Basic Tomato Sauce for dinner, and even chop the vegetables for the Roasted Mediterranean Vegetables side dish.

Day 2 of your Paleo Journey

After the successes of yesterday and a good intake of vitamins you may well be feeling a little more alert today and have woken up actually feeling hungry. If you come from a place of excess caffeine or refined starch consumption you might have a headache; take analgesia to get you through if you need it. Make sure that you drink plenty of water and snack on fruit or nuts if you get hungry.

Enjoy your meals -

BREAKFAST - Bacon and Mushroom Frittata; Roast Cherry Tomatoes
LUNCH - Chicken Salad with Olives and Artichokes
DINNER - Baked Fish with Tomato and Olives; Roasted Mediterranean Vegetables
DESSERT - Apple and Cinnamon Crunch

Nutrition - Fibre 100%+, Sodium 102%, Potassium 100%+, Iron 100%+. Magnesium 100%+, Vitamin A 100%+, Vitamin B12 100%+, Vitamin B6 100%+, Vitamin C 100%+, Vitamin D 1%, Vitamin E 100%+, Vitamin K 9%

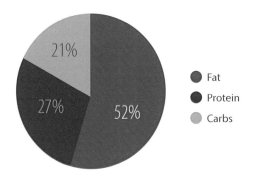

Exercise

A Swiss Ball is a cost effective way to introduce core strengthening into your daily routine. Use a Swiss Ball instead of a chair wherever possible and discover how quickly your posture improves. You will also need a Swiss Ball for the Tabata Transformation programme so this is good practice and a worthy investment.

Stress Management

Yesterday you looked at the sources of stress in your life. Today, take some time to consider how you react to these different stressors. Do you have different mechanisms for different sources of stress? Record your thoughts on how you react to stress. You may find it useful to start the Introduction to Yoga programme to help you identify and deal with triggers of stress in your everyday life.

Sleep

Don't forget that quality of sleep has a major impact upon every area of your life and consequently your health and weight loss goals. Today, consider setting up a bedtime routine that is conducive to sleep. Start with going to bed at the same time each night and getting up at the same time each morning; allowing for eight hours of sleep each night. Make a record, of how well you slept the night before.

Self-Awareness

Don't forget that self-awareness is the key to getting the most out of your life. This plan is all about doing something important for yourself; take the time today to consider how much you value yourself and prioritise your own self-worth. Record your thoughts.

Planning

What practical steps can you take today that will make life easier tomorrow? Not much kitchen prep required for tomorrow as long as you have Chicken Stock ready. If you eat lunch out of the house you will need to prepare the Thai Green Chicken Soup in advance.

Day 3 of your Paleo Journey

If you are going to suffer any detox symptoms, today will most likely be the day they kick in. If you need to, and are in a position to do so, take it easy. Everyone differs in this respect; you may find that gentle movement or fresh air helps or you may find that energy levels are so low that you simply need to rest.

The majority of individuals feel no untoward symptoms at all and you could well be bursting with energy. Regardless of how you feel mentally and physically you probably need some red meat proteins today, plenty of healthy fats and even a bit of comfort food; we have provided it all in today's menu and even included a restorative soup in case you feel a tad worse for wear.

Don't forget that right now your body's repair mechanisms have gone into overdrive, especially if you have lacked nutrients for quite some time. Make sure that you drink plenty of water and snack on fruit or nuts if you get hungry.

Enjoy your meals -

BREAKFAST - Scrambled Eggs with Smoked Salmon, Avocado and Dill
LUNCH - Thai Green Chicken Soup
DINNER - Steak with Garlic Mushrooms; Parsnip Fries; Spinach,
Apple and Fennel Salad

Nutrition - Fibre 100%+, Sodium 92%, Potassium 100%+, Iron 100%+, Magnesium 100%+, Vitamin A 23%, Vitamin B12 100%+, Vitamin B6 100%+, Vitamin C 33%+, Vitamin D 1%, Vitamin E 100%+, Vitamin K 17%

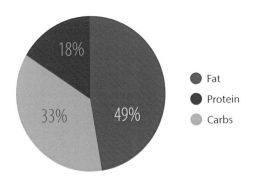

Exercise

Depending on your energy levels today you may benefit from some gentle stretching exercises; perhaps in the fresh air, weather permitting. Try this simple backstretch – kneeling on all fours, with hands shoulder width apart and back flat, let your head drop and arch your back upwards as if pulling your navel to your spine. Hold for 30 seconds and then reverse the movement, bringing your head up and pushing your navel towards the floor. Repeat five times. A great tension reliever and energiser. Alternatively, look up the cool down exercises in Tabata Transformation for a gentle stretching routine.

Stress Management

So far, you have looked at the sources of stress in your life and the ways in which you react to them. Consider how many of these sources could be removed from your life with simple techniques such as learning to prioritise, limiting contact with stressful people, and learning to say no. Record your thoughts on how you might eliminate some sources of stress.

Sleep

Don't forget that quality of sleep has a major impact upon every area of your life and consequently your health and weight loss goals. Still thinking about bedtime routines, are there ways that you could wind down at night that could be more relaxing than your current activities? Could you read a book in a quiet space instead of watching TV or move bath time to just before bed? Keep a record of how well you slept the night before.

Self-Awareness

Don't forget that self-awareness is the key to getting the most out of your life. Identify your strengths and weaknesses, considering how well you use them in your everyday life. Could you put your strengths to better use or seek help in areas that you are less adept at? Remember we are all good at something so we don't all need to be good at everything. Record your thoughts.

Planning

What practical steps can you take today that will make life easier tomorrow? If you eat lunch away from home you will need to make the Butternut, Sage and Walnut Soup in advance. Marinating the Tandoori Chicken two days in advance is a good idea.

Day 4 of your Paleo Journey

By now you should be hitting your stride as far as eating is concerned. If suffering from detox symptoms, you could still be feeling a bit shaky on your feet but the benefits of all those vegetables should be making their presence known with an increased sense of vitality and wellbeing. Energy could be low and/or you may be having difficulty sleeping as your body adjusts. Keep going with gentle exercise and movement (more if you feel capable) and remember to drink plenty of water to flush out those toxins. Snack on berries and nuts if you feel the need but the habit of reaching for snacks may begin to dissipate.

Enjoy your meals -

BREAKFAST - Bacon, Avocado and Tomato with Parsley and Walnut Oil
LUNCH - Butternut, Sage and Walnut Soup
DINNER - Turkey Puttanesca; Greens with Lemon, Olive Oil and Pine Nuts

Nutrition - Fibre 89%, Sodium 100%+, Potassium 93%, Iron 100%+, Magnesium 100%+, Vitamin A 54%, Vitamin B12 100%+, Vitamin B6 100%+, Vitamin C 100%+, Vitamin D 1%, Vitamin E 100%+, Vitamin K 11%

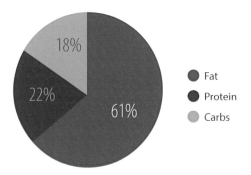

Exercise

Mixing it up is the key to exercising Paleo style and to function optimally your body requires perpetual movement. Sitting at a desk all day, or in front of the TV all evening contributes to modern diseases as much as poor diet. Aim to get up and move about every 30 minutes and place items in a room, like files or the remote, so that you constantly have to keep getting up. Set a reminder if you need to; there are even some useful apps on the market.

Stress Management

So far we have looked at stressors in your life and tried to identify any that could be avoided. But if a source of stress is impossible to remove then maybe there are ways to alter it? Maybe a compromise is the solution or perhaps you need to work on being more assertive? Record your thoughts on ways you could alter stressful situations.

Sleep

Don't forget that quality of sleep has a major impact upon every area of your life and consequently your health and weight loss goals. So far we have concentrated on building a routine but take some time today to consider your sleep environment also. Think about how comfortable your bed is; does your pillow offer enough support, or is your mattress past its best? Make a record each day of how well you slept the night before.

Self-Awareness

Don't forget that self-awareness is the key to getting the most out of your life. The ideas presented in this weekly planner are not intended to achieve vast sweeping changes in a week but are there to give you an idea of what is involved with a holistic approach to wellbeing. At the core stands reflection and it is one of the greatest tools for self-development. Practice reflection on a daily basis and it will soon become a normal part of everyday life; consider how you handled a certain event and explore ways in which you could improve the outcomes. Record your thoughts.

Planning

What practical steps can you take today that will make life easier tomorrow? If you eat lunch away from home you will need to prepare the Stuffed Turkey Rolls for tomorrow.

Day 5 of your Paleo Journey

Well, Friday is finally here and you have almost made it through the week. We hope that it has been a revelation rather than a chore and that you are really starting to feel the benefits; not to mention the shrinking waistline. You should be starting to feel an increase in energy and a difference in the way that your body perceives hunger; rather than cravings every few hours, accompanied by irritability, you should be experiencing discernible feelings of hunger that respond well to a balanced meal. With a decrease in cravings you should find that preparing food is a relaxing and enjoyable experience rather than an Olympic effort to get sustenance on the table.

Enjoy your meals -

BREAKFAST - Scrambled Eggs Piperade
LUNCH - Stuffed Turkey Rolls with Italian Vegetables; Spinach, Apple and Fennel Salad
DINNER - Tandoori Chicken; Sweet Potato and Spinach Curry; Greens with Lemon, Olive Oil and Pine Nuts
DESSERT - Baked Banana and Chocolate

Nutrition - Fibre 100%, Sodium 100%+, Potassium 100%+, Iron 100%+, Magnesium 100%+, Vitamin A 100%+, Vitamin B12 100%+, Vitamin B6 100%+, Vitamin C 61%, Vitamin D 1%, Vitamin E 100%+, Vitamin K 17%

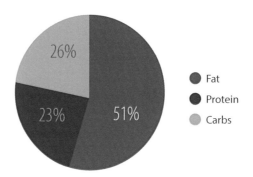

Exercise

Following on from yesterday and the theory of perpetual movement, invest in a pedometer to keep track of daily steps taken. The goal is 10,000 steps per day; a number that requires more conscious activity than most of us actually do. A pedometer is not an expensive item and there are many free apps that do the job just as well. If you have not suffered any side effects and are feeling the boost in energy you should be exploring the exercise programmes!

Stress Management

The next stage in dealing with life's stressors, if you can't avoid them or alter them, is learning to adapt. Reframing is a popular technique that after a while becomes second nature; try viewing the situation as part of the bigger picture or looking at things in a positive light. Record your thoughts on how you might practice reframing situations. This is covered in depth in *Paleo: 12 Weeks to Change Your Life*.

Sleep

Don't forget that quality of sleep has a major impact upon every area of your life and consequently your health and weight loss goals. Friday night could well be a late night with a lie in planned for Saturday morning but in order to get the most benefit from a sleep routine every effort should be made to stick to it seven days a week. Understandably this approach does not work for everyone but if you suffer from sleep issues it is a worthwhile consideration. Make a record each day of how well you slept the night before.

Self-Awareness

Don't forget that self-awareness is the key to getting the most out of your life. Practising mindfulness is a popular theory in weight loss practice but it can extend into every area of your life. To be mindful means to live in the moment and not drift through life completely unaware of your surroundings or actions. For the most part, our subconscious can take over and many actions become second nature. Take time to notice the details of your surroundings and consider your actions. Record your thoughts.

Planning

What practical steps can you take today that will make life easier tomorrow? If you are home over the weekend then you won't need to do any advance kitchen preparation today.

Day 6 of your Paleo Journey

If the beginning of your week was Monday, then the weekend has arrived and for many of you a chance to be at home and enjoy some leisure time. Whatever you enjoy doing with your weekend, take some time out to enjoy a leisurely breakfast and put your feet up at the end of the day with a delicious creamy hot chocolate.

Enjoy your meals -

BREAKFAST - Full English Stir Fry
LUNCH - Tandoori Chicken and Roasted Vegetable Wrap
DINNER - Beef Pot Roast
EVENING SNACK - Coconut Hot Chocolate

Nutrition - Fibre 100%+, Sodium 56%, Potassium 100%+, Iron 100%+, Magnesium 100%+, Vitamin A 100%+, Vitamin B12 100%+, Vitamin B6 100%+, Vitamin C 100%+, Vitamin D 1%, Vitamin E 100%+, Vitamin K 14%

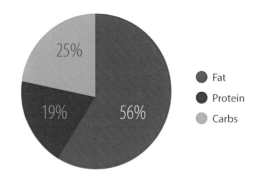

Exercise

You could make swimming a regular part of your routine; at the end of the week it can push aside the cobwebs and set you up with energy for the weekend ahead. Relaxing, muscle toning and invigorating, a relaxing swim could be just what you need. Make full use of the shower by taking some citrus essential oils and practise some dry body brushing before you get dressed. Pamper and exercise all in one go.

Stress Management

When all else fails, you may simply need to accept that not everything in life can be under your control. By dealing pro-actively with all sources of stress and finding alternative ways of dealing with them you pave the way for coping with the things that you cannot change. Record your thoughts on how you might learn to accept these things.

Sleep

Don't forget that quality of sleep has a major impact upon every area of your life and consequently your health and weight loss goals. Reassess how you have been sleeping this week and consider making some adjustments to your sleeping area. Are there any sources of light that could be affecting your quality of sleep? Eliminate sources of electronic light such a standby sensors or digital alarm clocks and invest in a pair of blackout blinds for the window; you may be surprised by how refreshed you feel in the morning when sleeping in a completely dark room. Make a record each day of how well you slept the night before.

Self-Awareness

Don't forget that self-awareness is the key to getting the most out of your life. Any schoolteacher will tell you that a healthy mind is an inquisitive one and there is no reason why that should stop once you leave school. If you don't keep asking questions then you have no reason to provide the answers. By constantly asking "why" of yourself and the world you are forced to explore endless possibilities. Try it; don't be satisfied with "I don't know".

Planning

What practical steps can you take today that will make life easier tomorrow? Tomorrow's breakfast requires Basic Tomato Sauce but there should be enough left from earlier in the week.

Day 7 of your Paleo Journey

Well, the final day of your seven day Paleo challenge is here and some of you will be feeling a spring in your step and have shed some of that excess weight. For those of you who have been through some detox symptoms, you may still feel a lack of energy but with a certain underlying vitality as your body heals itself; you may have experienced considerable weight loss as toxins are eliminated from fat cells. Use today to continue with the healthy eating plan, reflect on the week behind you and consider where you will go from here. Well done you.

Enjoy your meals -

BREAKFAST - Sausage and Egg Peperonata
LUNCH - Beef, Avocado and Spinach Salad with Coriander and Ginger Dressing
DINNER - Lamb Chops with Cumin and Mint; Cauliflower Couscous

Nutrition - Fibre 100%+, Sodium 72%, Potassium 100%+, Iron 100%+, Magnesium 27%, Vitamin A 100%+, Vitamin B12 100%+, Vitamin B6 100%+, Vitamin C 100%+, Vitamin D 1%, Vitamin E 100%+, Vitamin K 14%

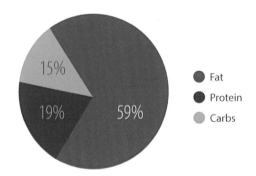

Exercise

Hopefully this final day of the plan coincides with Sunday or at least some down time in your schedule. With this day being all about reflecting on the week just gone and considering the months ahead, head outdoors into nature and take a long leisurely hike that will keep your body moving and help you think clearly.

Stress Management

After a week's crash course in some of the theory behind stress management, don't forget one last important factor; make room in your life for the things that you enjoy. Nurturing yourself is of utmost importance and yours by right, not because you have earned it. Make time each day to go for a walk, soak in a bath or read a book. Record any thoughts.

Sleep

Don't forget that quality of sleep has a major impact upon every area of your life and consequently your health and weight loss goals. We have covered many of the areas of sleep management that can improve the quality of your sleep but you may find that your dietary change this week has had an impact on your sleep. You could experiment with making changes to the time that you eat your evening meal or many find that they respond well to a magnesium supplement at night. Make a record each day of how well you slept the night before.

Self-Awareness

Don't forget that self-awareness is the key to getting the most out of your life. We put great store in our rituals; they provide familiarity and comfort in an often uncertain world. But it can be easy to get stuck in a rut and miss out on the many opportunities for a different experience or viewpoint. Make a point of trying new things and seeing the world from another angle. It can be as simple as sitting in a different chair at the dinner table or something bigger like never turning down an invitation (whether it is lunch or white water rafting).

SECTION 11
Congratulations

You have made it to the end of your 7 day Paleo plan. Congratulations. You have taken the first step towards a healthy and sustainable lifestyle by choosing to take control of your life. We hope that this will not be the end but the start of your Paleo journey.

Take time to record your thoughts and achievements throughout the past week, reflecting on the good as well as the bad. You will hopefully not have suffered from any side effects and will be feeling refreshed and full of energy. If you have felt the impact of the detox to your system then be proud of yourself for sticking at it. We promise that it will be worth it. Your body is taking its first steps towards wellbeing and you will be amazed at the results that you can achieve.

We hope that the daily lifestyle and coaching tips have helped to provide some clarity on the stress triggers in your life and how controlling these can dramatically improve your health and wellbeing. If you have not done so already you should read Introduction to Yoga. This will not only help you to identify the sources of stress but also provides a mechanism as to how to deal with the stresses of everyday life. This is also discussed further in Paleo: 12 Weeks to Change Your Life.

If you have not been able to incorporate exercise into your 7 day plan then we recommend that you start to now introduce this into your weekly routine. You will achieve the best results from combining Paleo with an exercise plan and you will be shocked at just how good it will make you feel. If you have not done so already then you should read Tabata Transformation. This will provide you with the most effective exercise programme to compliment your new Paleo lifestyle. Give it a try. It will change how you exercise forever and will provide incredible results.

Remember that this is just the beginning. You have an exciting journey ahead of you that will lead to the healthy and sustainable lifestyle that many dream of and only few make the transition to forever. You need to build upon the momentum from this week and take this forward to complete the 12 Week Plan provided in Paleo: 12 Weeks to Change Your Life.

This is the time that it takes to truly change behaviour and for it to become habit forming. Once you have completed the 12 week programme you will be equipped both physically and mentally to make intuitive decisions to maintain a truly sustainable lifestyle.

Everything you need to move forward is set out in Paleo: 12 Weeks to Change Your Life and will develop upon what you have learnt in your 7 day plan and will run alongside Tabata Transformation and Introduction to Yoga to provide you with the most outstanding results.

Make a commitment and don't look back

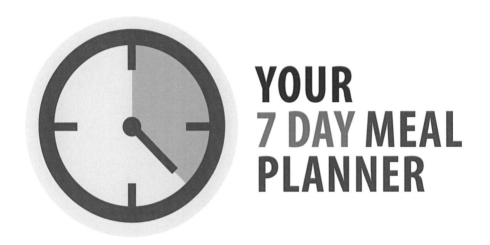

YOUR
7 DAY MEAL
PLANNER

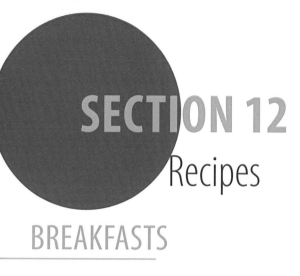

SECTION 12
Recipes

BREAKFASTS

Eating plenty of protein at breakfast is one of the best ways to accelerate weightloss. If you are used to toast, cereal or some kind of bar or biscuit on the run, then breakfast can be the trickiest part of Paleo to get used to. Many Paleo followers eat plates of vegetables or leftover dinner for breakfast as it is easy and nutritious but we have designed a range of breakfast dishes that shouldn't feel too unfamiliar. It may take more time to prepare and eat but you will banish those mid-morning cravings and sugar dips for good.

Sausage and Egg Peperonata
R E C I P E

A soft chunky sauce of peppers and onions is added to sausages and topped with eggs. Baked in the oven, it makes a delicious and satisfying breakfast dish.

Servings: 2

Preparation Time: 10 minutes

Cooking Time: 50 minutes

Total Time: 1 hour

Ingredients

2 red peppers, thinly sliced

2 onions, thinly sliced

$^1/_2$ recipe Basic Tomato Sauce (in the extras section)

1 tbsp extra virgin olive oil

4 sausages

4 eggs

Fresh parsley for garnish

Freshly ground black pepper

Procedure

1. Preheat the oven to 180°C.

2. Bake the sausages in the oven for about 20-30 minutes until cooked through.

3. Heat the olive oil in a large pan over a medium heat.

4. Add onions and peppers with salt and pepper, then cook for about 10 minutes. You want it to soften but not colour.

5. Turn the heat down a little, add the tomato sauce, and cook for about 20 minutes until it is thick and glossy.

6. When everything is ready cut the sausages into chunks, mix into the Peperonata and place in an ovenproof dish.

7. Make wells in the mixture to take the eggs. Crack an egg into each hole and bake in the oven for roughly 10 minutes.

8. The white should be set and the yolk still runny.

9. Serve hot from the oven, with chopped fresh parsley strewn over the top.

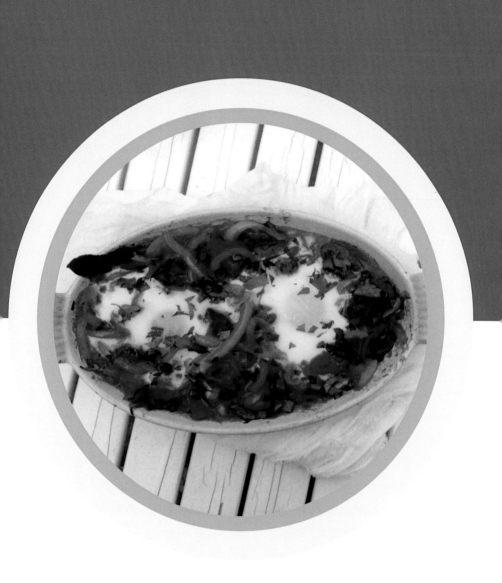

Bacon and Mushroom Frittata

This dish is great served cold and makes a handy stand in for a lunch time sandwich; you may need to finish the top under the grill before the bottom gets overly browned. Goes well with Roast Tomatoes and Herbs.

Servings: 2

Preparation Time: 10 minutes

Cooking Time: 30 minutes

Total Time: 40 minutes

Ingredients

6 large free range eggs, beaten

4 rashers free range bacon, diced

4 large mushrooms, sliced

1 pinch freshly ground black pepper

1 tbsp fresh parsley, chopped

1 tbsp olive oil

Procedure

1. Heat the oil in a non-stick frying pan over a medium heat and fry the bacon with the mushrooms until cooked through.

2. Beat the eggs with the herbs and seasoning and pour into the frying pan.

3. Turn the heat down and cook for as long as you can without the base burning. If the top doesn't set quickly finish the frittata under the grill.

4. Serve in slices; either hot or cold

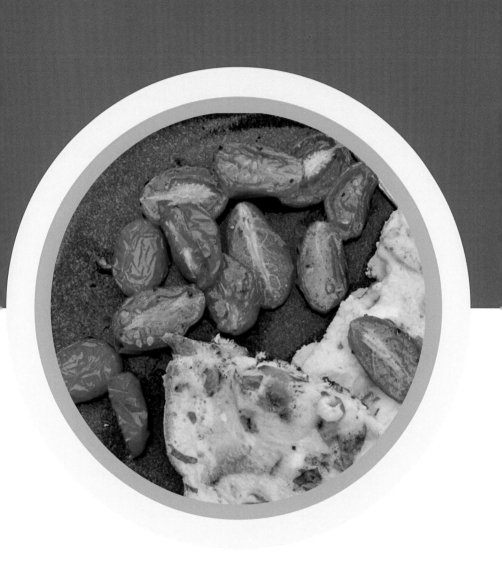

Scrambled Eggs with Smoked Salmon, Avocado and Dill

Smoked salmon with scrambled eggs is a classic breakfast dish; here we add soft avocado for extra nutrition and flavour, plus a snip of fresh dill. Take the eggs from the heat as soon as they begin to set; there is no dairy here to keep it soft so cooking well is vital.

Servings: 2

Preparation Time: 10 minutes

Cooking Time: 2 minutes

Total Time: 12 minutes

Ingredients

4 large eggs, beaten

100g smoked salmon, chopped

2 ripe avocado, chopped

1 tsp fresh dill, finely chopped

1 tbsp olive oil

Procedure

1.   Place a saucepan over a medium heat and warm the oil.

2.   Add the eggs and stir until set.

3.   Remove from the heat and stir in the salmon, avocado and dill.

4.   Eat whilst hot.

Scrambled Eggs Piperade

RECIPE

A play on a classic Basque dish these vibrant spicy scrambled eggs make an excellent breakfast for days when you are short on time and need a little push. If you have never considered chilli and garlic at breakfast then now could be the time to change your mind. The chillies stimulate appetite and get the metabolism going as well as waking up all your senses; garlic is also great for a sluggish system.

Servings: 2

Preparation Time: 10 minutes

Cooking Time: 10 minutes

Total Time: 20 minutes

Ingredients

6 large free range eggs

1 garlic clove, crushed

1 red chilli pepper, finely chopped

1 tsp smoked paprika

1 tbsp olive oil

1 pinch sea salt

2 tbsp fresh parsley, finely chopped

Procedure

1. Heat the oil in a medium sized pan over a low heat and add all of the ingredients.

2. Stir slowly whilst the eggs slowly set and combine with the flavourings.

3. As soon as the eggs reach setting point, stir in the parsley and serve immediately.

4. Eat hot as soon as they are ready.

Spinach, Pepper and Mushroom Omelette

RECIPE

A good omelette for breakfast is the mainstay of the Paleo diet and will keep you going right up until lunch. Use the freshest, free range eggs that you can find and do not beat them until just before you need them. A touch of paprika added to the mix enlivens the flavours and wakes up the taste buds.

Servings: 2

Preparation Time: 10 minutes

Cooking Time: 10 minutes

Total Time: 20 minutes

Ingredients

4 large eggs, beaten

6 mushrooms, sliced

1 red pepper, thinly sliced

2 handfuls baby spinach leaves

1 tbsp olive oil

1 pinch sea salt

1 pinch black pepper

1 pinch paprika

Procedure

1. Heat a non-stick frying pan over a medium heat and add the oil.

2. Gently fry the mushrooms and pepper until the pepper is soft and wilting. Add the spinach and cook until it has wilted down. Tip the filling onto a plate.

3. Beat the eggs together with the seasonings.

4. Add the eggs and scrape the sides into the middle, using a spatula, letting the runny eggs fill the spaces that you create.

5. Continue until the egg is almost set.

6. Add the filling on top and fold one half over.

7. Cut in half and serve on two plates.

8. Eat immediately.

Full English Stir Fry

One of the perks of Paleo is getting to keep your cooked breakfast. This version is slightly different as it is all cooked together in one pan. Feel free to introduce peppers, herbs or any other vibrant flavours into the mix; you would be surprised what works.

Servings: 2

Preparation Time: 10 minutes

Cooking Time: 20 minutes

Total Time: 30 minutes

Ingredients

200g mushrooms, sliced

1 red onion, sliced

2 large tomatoes, chopped

2 Paleo friendly pork sausages, chopped

4 rashers back bacon, chopped

2 eggs

1 tbsp olive oil

A good twist of black pepper

Procedure

1. Fry the onion first in a little of the olive oil and then add the mushrooms with a good twist of black pepper.

2. Once the mushrooms begin to break down and cook, add the sausage. Cook for about 5 to 10 minutes until the sausage is thoroughly cooked then add the bacon.

3. Once the bacon is cooked, add the tomatoes and crack the eggs over the top, turning the heat down low.

4. When the eggs are set you can plate up and enjoy a good breakfast.

Bacon, Avocado and Tomato with Parsley and Walnut Oil

The calorie density and nutritional value of avocado cannot be underestimated when you are eating Paleo, especially in the early stages when you may not be getting enough calories. Eaten for breakfast the world over, avocado is an essential addition to your breakfast repertoire. This breakfast salad is useful for when you are on the go as it transports well and particularly good if you are feeling a little tired. If you have cooked bacon and hard boiled eggs ready in the fridge at all times it becomes even easier.

Servings: 2

Preparation Time: 10 minutes

Cooking Time: 10 minutes

Total Time: 20 minutes

Ingredients

4 rashers cooked back bacon, chopped

1 ripe avocado, chopped

4 hardboiled eggs, chopped

2 large ripe tomatoes, chopped

1 tbsp walnut oil

2 tbsp fresh parsley, chopped

Procedure

1.   Mix all of the ingredients together and eat when you like.

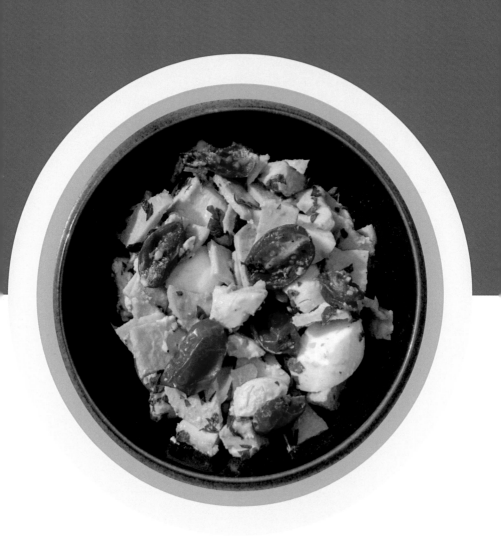

LUNCH

Often eaten out of the house, lunch can be tricky if you don't prepare for it. Salads, with dressings and fragile ingredients packed separately, can be easily boxed up, whilst soup can be heated in an office microwave. Bread sandwiches can be replaced by lettuce wraps, and making extra portions of cooked meats you can save time in the kitchen. Using leftovers is the best way to economise in the kitchen; as well as reducing food waste.

Chicken Salad with Olives and Artichokes

RECIPE

Use leftover cooked chicken to make a salad bursting with flavours and textures. If you are taking this as a pack lunch, pack leaves and dressing separately to add before eating. The artichokes and olives add something a little special to the basic salad; try to find those packed in olive oil without any extra additions.

Servings: 2

Preparation Time: 10 minutes

Total Time: 10 minutes

Ingredients

300g leftover cooked chicken

100g mixed salad leaf

2 large ripe tomatoes, chopped

$1/_2$ cucumber, chopped

2 apples, chopped

6 spring onions, finely chopped

12 pieces deli style artichokes

20 Kalamata olives

20 raw almonds

2 tbsp olive oil

1 tbsp balsamic vinegar

2 tbsp fresh chopped parsley

Freshly ground black pepper

Procedure

1. Layer all the ingredients and toss together with salt, oil and vinegar immediately prior to serving.

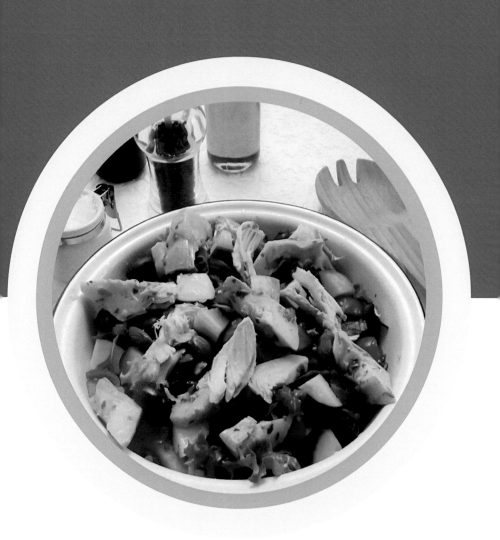

Thai Green Chicken Soup

RECIPE

This recipe uses fresh Chicken Stock but you could use good quality ready-made stock if you wish; make sure to check the label first. Thai green paste is not difficult to make and is far superior to the kind in jars as even a good quality paste will lose its vibrancy; make double and freeze it for next time. A really soothing dish that will lift flagging spirits and energise a tired body, this is a must have during that first week of clean eating and we have hopefully timed it for exactly the right moment. It re-heats well so can easily be transported if necessary. Ingredients shouldn't be too hard to source nowadays; look for the best quality freeze dried lime leaves that you can find.

Servings: 2

Preparation Time: 10 minutes

Cooking Time: 10 minutes

Total Time: 20 minutes

Ingredients

For the curry paste

1 bunch fresh coriander

4 red chillies

4 stalks lemongrass

2 inches ginger

4 cloves garlic

4 shallots

2 tsp ground cumin

1 tsp ground coriander

2 limes, juice only

For the soup

1 tbsp coconut oil

400ml chicken stock

200g coconut milk

6 lime leaves

1 bunch fresh basil (Thai if you can get it)

200g leftover Lemon and Sage Roast Chicken

Procedure

1. Blitz all of the paste ingredients in a food processor until you have a coarse paste. It seems quite fibrous but suits the final dish.

2. Freeze half of your paste and set the rest aside.

3. Heat the coconut oil in a saucepan over a medium heat and fry the paste for a minute or so.

4. Now add the coconut milk, stock and lime leaves. Allow it to simmer gently for about 5 minutes.

5. Add the cooked chicken and fresh basil before serving hot.

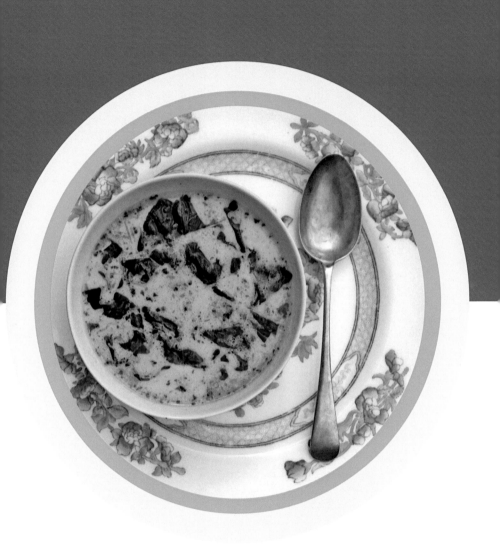

Tandoori Chicken and Roasted Vegetable Wrap

Again you are using leftovers for lunch which is not only economical but makes good use of ingredients and cooking time too. This time we are using the Mediterranean Vegetables and leftover Tandoori Chicken to create a lettuce parcel. The concept of lettuce Paleo wraps is not a new one and the final shape depends on the lettuce you have. We used young Romaine lettuce and piled the filling on top to create a crunchy scoop. With bigger leaves or iceberg lettuce you can wrap the filling inside to make an ad-hoc sandwich.

Servings: 2

Preparation Time: 10 minutes

Total Time: 10 minutes

Ingredients

8 large Romaine lettuce leaves

200g Leftover Tandoori Chicken, chopped

150g Roast Mediterranean Vegetables

2 tbsp fresh coriander, chopped

2 tbsp fresh mint, chopped

Procedure

1. Mix the chicken with the vegetables and herbs.

2. Pile onto the lettuce leaves and eat with your hands.

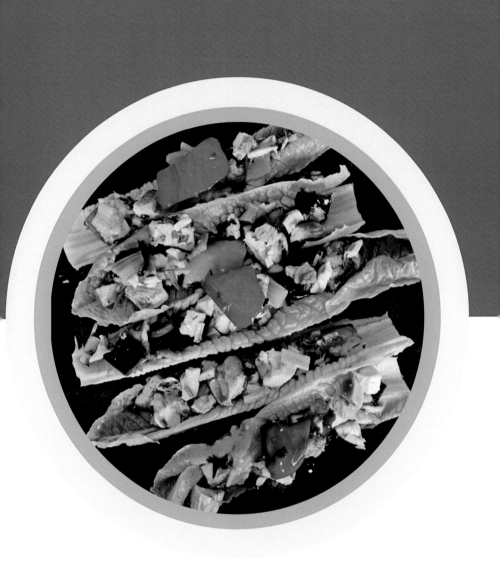

Mackerel Nicoise

RECIPE

This salad is very good slightly warm but will eat just as well cold if you want a packed lunch for work. Blanched green beans with just a little squeaky bite are added to plump smoked mackerel and sharp spring onions then tossed with a mustard dill dressing. We haven't included any eggs as mackerel is heavy enough by itself. But you are free to add this if you wish!

Servings: 2

Preparation Time: 15 minutes

Cooking Time: 5 minutes

Total Time: 20 minutes

Ingredients

2 mackerel fillets

1 bunch spring onions, chopped

200g fine green beans

12 black olives

For the dressing

2 tbsp fresh dill, chopped

1 tbsp balsamic vinegar

2 tbsp olive oil

1 tsp Dijon mustard

Freshly ground black pepper

Procedure

1. Bring a pan of salted water up to a rolling boil. Top and tail the green beans and then blanch them in the boiling water for about 5 minutes. Remove with a slotted spoon and plunge them into icy water if eating cold.

2. Make the dressing by whisking (or shaking in a jar) together the vinegar, oil, mustard, and pepper.

3. Toss the salad ingredients together with the dressing. If eating warm, heat the mackerel in a pan or in the microwave for just a few minutes until warmed through.

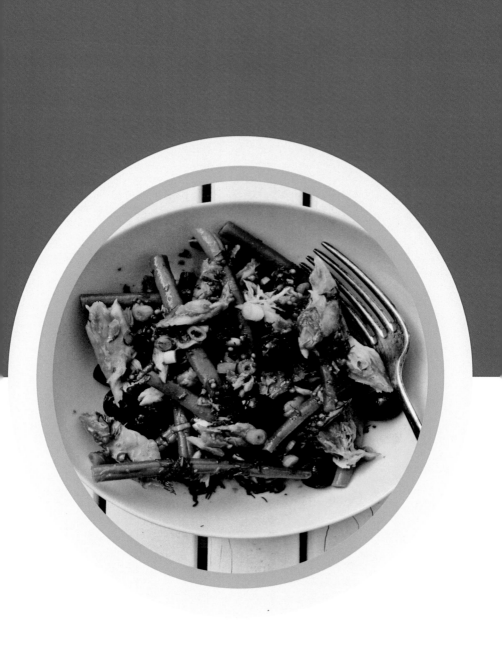

Butternut, Sage and Walnut Soup

A filling, smooth and comforting soup that you can make with water or fresh Chicken Stock. Homemade chicken stock is best, but you can use a high quality ready made one as long as you check the label for any nasties. The robust flavour of coconut oil suits the soup, and if you are feeling less than great you can add some block coconut cream for extra calories and richness. Use fresh sage if you can get it, otherwise dried is fine. Only use a little as sage can be very overpowering.

Servings: 4

Preparation Time: 15 minutes

Cooking Time: 30 minutes

Total Time: 45 minutes

Ingredients

1 large butternut squash, peeled and cubed

1 large onion coarsely chopped

1 small clove garlic, crushed

2 tbsp coconut oil

1 pinch sea salt

1 tsp paprika

1 tbsp lemon juice

300ml Chicken Stock (or water)

25g walnuts

1 tbsp fresh sage leaves (or 1 tsp dried)

Procedure

1. Heat the coconut oil in a large saucepan over a medium heat. Add the butternut, garlic, onion and salt. Stir to combine and cook gently for 5 to 10 minutes until everything begins to soften.

2. Add the paprika, stir to combine and pour in the cold stock.

3. Cook the soup gently until the butternut is soft and remove from the heat.

4. Blitz the soup in a processor until smooth, add the lemon juice and check the seasoning.

5. Chop the walnuts together with the sage to form a crunchy topping for the soup.

6. Serve hot with a sprinkle of topping and a slick of olive oil. Add a few chopped chillies if you like your food hot.

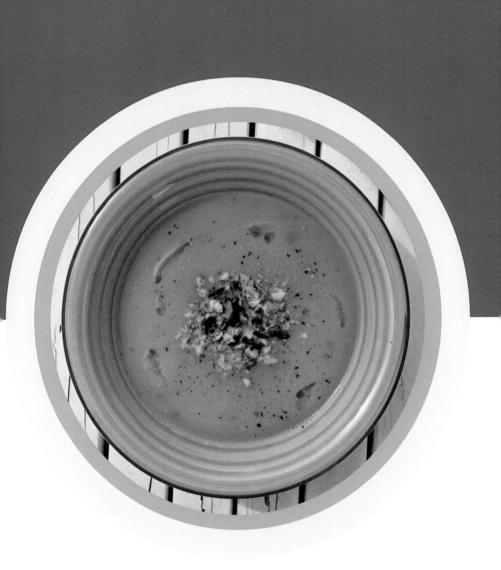

Stuffed Turkey Rolls
with Italian Vegetables

You can either use good quality cooked turkey breast from the deli counter or cook your own escalopes. If using raw escalopes, the stuffing is rolled inside and then cooked so the roll stays put. Turkey is a cost effective protein option and wonderfully versatile. The filling is made of leftover Roasted Mediterranean Vegetables with artichoke, olives and basil added. The recipe uses raw turkey; if you want to use cooked turkey just make up the filling, roll and go. You can buy raw turkey escalopes (which are essentially slices of breast meat) or buy breast and slice it yourself. Don't worry if they look too thick; you are going to flatten it with a frying pan.

Servings: 2

Preparation Time: 15 minutes

Cooking Time: 15 minutes

Total Time: 30 minutes

Ingredients

300g turkey breast steaks

For the filling

150g Roast Mediterranean Vegetables

75g artichoke hearts, chopped

75g Kalamata olives, sliced

10 basil leaves, torn

Procedure

1. Preheat the oven to 200°C.

2. First, you need to flatten the escalopes. Place one turkey steak between two pieces of cling film and hit it hard with the flat base of a frying pan. Peel away the cling film and you should be left with a thin turkey escalope. Do them all.

3. Mix the vegetables with the olives, artichokes and basil.

4. Divide the mixture between the escalopes, arranging it in a line across the centre of each. Roll up the escalopes and place on a greased baking tray.

5. Bake until the turkey is cooked; about 15 minutes should do it.

6. You can eat these hot or pack them cold for a lunch at work. They work well cold as the meat and filling create a self-contained parcel when cool.

Beef, Avocado and Spinach Salad with Coriander and Ginger Dressing

A fresh and filling salad with a vibrant dressing to bring life to tired taste buds. Using the leftover beef from the pot roast is good kitchen economics and makes sense in terms of both time and money. When doing a weekly shop as so many of us do (it is not always practical to visit the greengrocers twice a week) the key is to use up what you buy in as many ways as you can. Keeping salads small and simple with just a few ingredients ensures that there is always plenty of variety.

Servings: 2

Preparation Time: 15 minutes

Total Time: 15 minutes

Ingredients

300g cooked leftover beef, chopped or sliced

120g baby leaf spinach

1 ripe avocado, chopped

2 tbsp olive oil

$^1/_2$ lemon, juice only

1 inch fresh ginger, grated

2 tbsp fresh coriander, chopped

1 red chilli, chopped (optional)

1 pinch sea salt

1 pinch freshly ground black pepper

2 tbsp sesame seeds, toasted

Procedure

1. Toss all of the ingredients together and serve. There is no need to mix dressing separately, although if you are taking this for lunch at work you will want to carry the dressing in a small tub. Avocados are also best cut immediately prior to eating.

DINNER

Dinner, especially during the working week, often needs to be quick and easy to prepare. That said, once your insulin levels are back under control you won't be walking in the house ready to eat the contents of the fridge and too tired to function. Entering the kitchen relaxed and ready to engage with the preparation of delicious healthy food is part of the joy of Paleo cooking. Some recipes need longer than others so perhaps keep these for the times when you have longer to prepare; think about leftovers and where they might fit into the next day's lunch.

Turkey Puttanesca
RECIPE

This recipe uses your Basic Tomato Sauce recipe, with added anchovies, olives and chilli. Added to stir fried turkey breast it makes a flavourful and satisfying meal. We serve it with filling and delicious greens with the extra crunch of pinenuts.

Servings: 2

Preparation Time: 15 minutes

Cooking Time: 20 minutes

Total Time: 35 minutes

Ingredients

400g turkey breast, cut into strips

1 tbsp olive oil

$^1/_3$ recipe Basic Tomato Sauce (in the extras section)

20 Kalamata olives

1 small tin anchovies, chopped

2 red chillies, finely chopped or whole

2 tbsp fresh parsley, chopped

Procedure

1. Heat the oil in a frying pan over a medium heat. Add the turkey strips and stir fry for a few minutes.

2. There are a few ways that you can now add the chilli. If you want a little subtle heat, pierce the chillies and add them whole to the pan. If you want more heat, add the chopped chillies to the turkey now.

3. Add the tomato sauce, anchovies and olives, give it a good stir and leave it to simmer over a low heat for about 15 to 20 minutes.

4. Serve hot with Greens, Lemon, Olive Oil and Pine Nuts for a full Italian flavour.

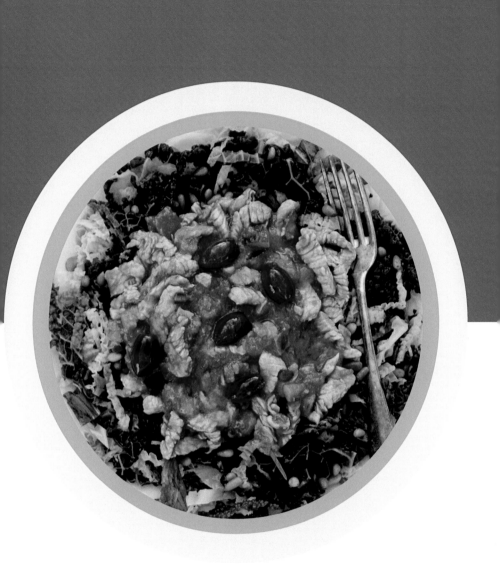

Steak with Garlic Mushrooms

Steak is absolutely great on a Paleo diet, filling you with energy and red muscle meat power. There are many people who think that a Paleo diet consists of large chunks of meat at each meal and far more steak than is affordable or good for you; nothing could be further from the truth.

Servings: 2

Preparation Time: 5 minutes

Cooking Time: 15 minutes

Total Time: 20 minutes

Ingredients

2 sirloin steaks (nice thick ones please, of the best quality you can afford)

1 tbsp olive oil

8 mushrooms, thinly sliced

2 cloves garlic, crushed

2 tbsp fresh parsley, chopped

Procedure

1. First, you need to bring the steaks to room temperature.

2. You oil the steak, not the pan. Rub each steak with a little of the oil, reserving the rest for the mushrooms, and season with pepper only.

3. Heat a large frying pan, preferably not non-stick as it does awful things to meat, until it is smoking hot.

4. As soon as you are ready to cook, salt the side that will touch the pan first. Lay both steaks, salt side down, in the hot pan and then leave it alone.

5. Your average steak should take roughly 2 minutes on each side for rare, 3 for medium or 4 for well done.

6. After the first timing is up, salt the upper surface of the steak and then flip the steaks over. Cook for the rest of the allotted time and then transfer to a hot plate to rest whilst you do the mushrooms.

7. Using the same pan, add the rest of the olive oil and the mushrooms. Season with salt and pepper, and cook quickly until they cook down and begin to brown. Turn the heat off, add the garlic and parsley then spoon the mushrooms over the steaks. You need to work quickly so that the garlic does not burn in the hot pan.

8. Serve the steaks with Parsnip Fries and Spinach, Fennel and Apple Salad.

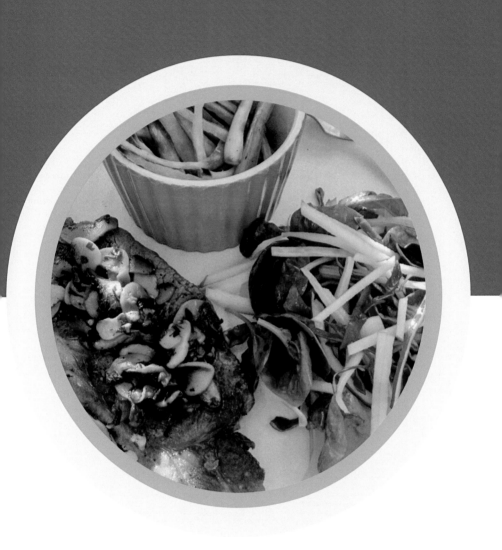

Lemon and Sage Roast Chicken

This chicken not only makes a delicious and satisfying meal but is the basis of several other meals too. We prefer roasting small chickens, and obviously the total time will depend on the size of your chickens; ours were about 1kg each and left in the oven for 90 minutes became tender and succulent. Cooking them breast side down keeps the flesh moist; turn over for the last 20 minutes to brown the skin on the breast. Small chickens like this will give you half a bird each for dinner, bones for stock, chicken for a gorgeous salad and cold cuts for the fridge to eat if you get hungry. And the best bit? You get to eat the skin.

Servings: 4

Preparation Time: 10 minutes

Cooking Time: 1 hour and 30 minutes

Total Time: 1 hour and 40 minutes

Ingredients

2 small roasting chickens

$^1/_2$ bunch sage leaves

1 large lemon

1 tbsp olive oil

1 pinch sea salt

Freshly ground black pepper

Procedure

1. Preheat the oven to 180C.

2. Rub the chickens all over with oil, salt and pepper. Place half of the sage and half a lemon in each cavity and place upside down in a roasting tray.

3. Roast the chickens for about 90 minutes (this is quite a slow temperature for roasting) until the leg pulls away from the rest of the bird with ease.

4. Turn over for 20 minutes to brown the skin, turning the oven temperature up if need be.

5. Leave the chickens to rest for 15 minutes before serving with Root Mash with Paprika and Fennel Seed.

Baked Fish with Tomato and Olives

A quick and easy fish dish for a light yet satisfying supper. You can buy fresh fish or make use of frozen fish fillets which are often far more economical; check the label to make sure that all it contains is fish. The chunkier the fillets, the better. It doesn't have to be cod; look for other types of fish with a firm white flake; you could even use salmon. This recipe makes use of the Basic Tomato Sauce that you have already prepped and cooks quickly in the oven.

Servings: 2

Preparation Time: 10 minutes

Cooking Time: 20 minutes

Total Time: 30 minutes

Ingredients

400g fish fillets

1 tbsp olive oil

$1/_3$ recipe Basic Tomato Sauce (in the extras section)

20 Kalamata olives

2 tbsp fresh parsley, chopped

Freshly ground black pepper

2 tbsp sesame seeds, toasted

Procedure

1. Preheat the oven to 200C.

2. Pour the oil into the bottom of an ovenproof dish and lay in the fish fillets.

3. Cover the fish with the sauce, scatter with olives and bake for roughly 20 minutes until the fish is completely opaque and flakes easily with a fork.

4. Scatter the fillets with the parsley and serve hot with your choice of side dishes.

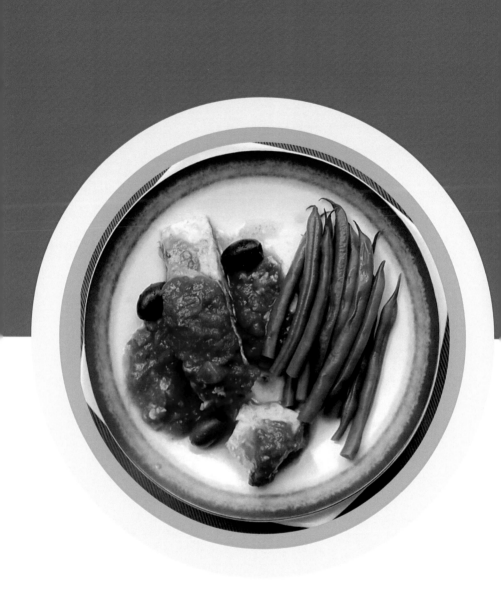

Lamb Chops with Cumin and Mint

RECIPE

Tender loin chops with their sweet meat and generous layer of fat crisp up beautifully in a hot oven and take nothing to prepare. Bringing them to room temperature first makes for a shorter cooking time and particularly tender meat. These chops with their slightly exotic hint of Eastern promise go well with the Cauliflower Couscous recipe.

Servings: 2

Preparation Time: 10 minutes

Cooking Time: 20 minutes

Total Time: 30 minutes

Ingredients

4 lamb chops

1 tbsp olive oil

1 tsp ground cumin

1 tbsp fresh mint, chopped

1 pinch sea salt

Freshly ground black pepper

Procedure

1. Preheat the oven to 180C and allow the chops to come up to room temperature.

2. Rub the chops all over with the oil, pepper, cumin and mint, and place in a roasting tin.

3. When you are ready to cook, sprinkle a little salt over the meat and place the chops in the oven.

4. Cook for about 20 minutes, turning once, until the meat is tender and the fat nice and brown.

5. Serve with Cauliflower Couscous.

Tandoori Chicken

This chicken is best marinated several days in advance; 24 hrs minimum should do it. You could use a ready-made spice paste; but you need to check that it does not contain wheat, preservatives or highly processed oils. We have included the recipe for a homemade spice blend that you can follow if you wish and have the spices to hand. Freshly ground spices are always best and a skill well worth acquiring if you are serious about changing your eating habits. If you can, get the butcher to spatchcock your chicken or, if you know how to, do this yourself. Otherwise, just keep the chickens whole, or use portions (include bone in breast if you can). The leftover chicken is used in a lunchtime recipe and makes plenty of cold cuts for the fridge.

Servings: 4
Preparation Time: 30 minutes
Cooking Time: 1 hour and 30 minutes
Inactive Time: 48 hours
Total Time: 50 hours

Ingredients

2 small roasting chickens, or equivalent
4 tbsp tandoori paste or homemade as below
For the tandoori paste
2 tsp coriander seed (ground or whole)
2 tsp cumin seed (ground or whole)
1 tsp fenugreek seed (ground or whole)
2 tsp black peppercorns (ground or whole)

$1/_4$ tsp cloves (ground or whole)
$1/_4$ tsp cardamom pods (ground or whole)
2 tsp paprika
2 tbsp olive oil
4 cloves garlic, crushed
4 hot green chillies, finely diced
2 inches ginger, grated

Procedure

1. Make slits all over the chicken so that the flavour can fully penetrate the flesh and rub all of the spice paste in well.

2. Cover with cling film and leave in the fridge for at least 24 hours.

3. When ready to cook, preheat the oven to 180C and lift the chicken from the marinade into a roasting tray.

4. If you have 2 small chickens, cook for roughly 90 minutes until the legs pull away easily from the body. If you are using portions you will need to alter the cooking time accordingly.

5. Sere the chicken hot with Spinach and Sweet Potato Curry and Greens with Lemon, Olive Oil and Pine Nuts. Leave the rest of the chicken for eating cold and quick lunches.

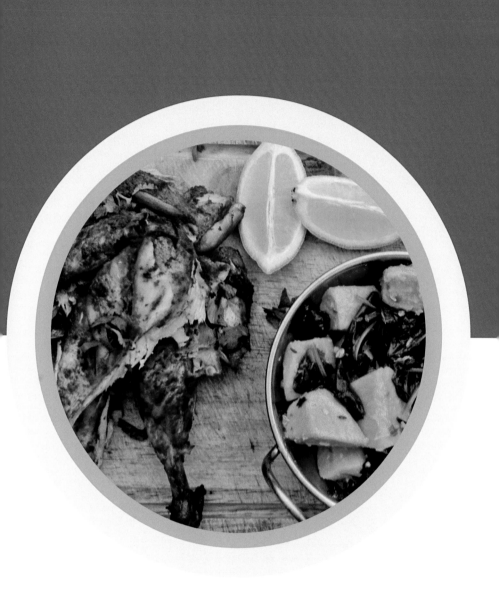

Beef Pot Roast

RECIPE

This is a dish for a day at home. It takes absolutely no effort at all but does need a good few hours in the oven. Choose a suitable cut for pot roasting with plenty of fat so it doesn't dry out and a good selection of root vegetables so that you need not prepare anything else. A big enough piece of meat ensures there is plenty left over for extra meals.

Servings: 2

Preparation Time: 30 minutes

Cooking Time: 2 hours

Total Time: 2 hours and 30 minutes

Ingredients

1 tbsp olive oil

750g silverside or brisket beef joint

6 carrots, chopped in large chunks

2 onions, quartered

2 leeks, chopped in large chunks

2 large parsnips, chopped in large chunks

1 small swede, chopped into large chunks

2 bay leaves

2 parsley sprigs

2 thyme sprigs

1 tbsp black peppercorns

3 cloves garlic

1 litre water

Sea salt

Procedure

1. Preheat the oven to 150C.

2. Place a large roasting tray over a medium heat and add the olive oil. Add the meat and the rest of the ingredients apart from the water and salt.

3. Brown everything all over, turning occasionally for an even colour. Once browned, remove from the hob and add the water with the salt.

4. Cover with tin foil and cook in the oven for about 2 hours or until the meat is fall apart tender.

5. Serve hot in thick slices with the vegetables and pan juices.

SIDES

Vegetable cookery, for all those delicious side dishes, is considered by many to be the trickiest area of cookery. Vegetables are in fact one of the simplest foods to cook and with a little attention to detail can be the star of the show. Try to keep it simple with a few key ingredients; that way you benefit from simpler flavours and greater scope for variety.

Parsnip Fries

R E C I P E

If you have duck or goose fat, it makes really good parsnip fries. If not, use olive oil. Whilst not a direct substitute for chips made with potatoes you may be surprised how well they actually go with a steak and crunchy salad. Cut them as thin as you can; you may burn a few skinny ends that way but you get a crisper finish. Lots of good sea salt is a must. You can also use sweet potatoes in this recipe instead of parsnips or why not try combining the two?

Servings: 2

Preparation Time: 15 minutes

Cooking Time: 20 minutes

Total Time: 35 minutes

Ingredients

3 large parsnips, cut into skinny fries

1 tbsp duck fat (or olive oil)

1 pinch sea salt

Procedure

1. Preheat the oven to 200C.

2. Put the duck fat on a roasting tray and place in the oven to heat.

3. When sizzling add the parsnips, stir to coat them in oil, sprinkle with salt and put the tray back in the oven.

4. Bake until crisp and golden; about 20 minutes depending on size and serve piping hot.

Spinach, Apple and Fennel Salad

This lovely crunchy salad pairs the robust green flavour of baby spinach and sweetens it with crunchy fresh apple. Red cabbage brings extra crunch and the anise tones of fennel elevate it into something special. A refreshing side dish that goes particularly well with Parsnip Fries and Garlic Mushroom Steak, this salad is a master class in using a few simple ingredients rather than throwing the salad compartment at the bowl.

Servings: 2

Preparation Time: 15 minutes

Total Time: 15 minutes

Ingredients

75g baby spinach leaves

$1/_4$ red cabbage, shredded

1 bulb young fennel, shredded

2 crisp green apples, finely sliced

1 tbsp walnut oil

2 tsp balsamic vinegar

1 pinch sea salt

Procedure

1. Toss ingredients together and serve.

Roast Tomatoes with Herbs

RECIPE

These tomatoes are not sun dried, or even mi-cuit, they are simply roasted tomatoes that work well hot or cold as a side dish. Roasting them in a hot oven with a little olive oil, salt and herbs softens them a little and really maximises the flavour. Make plenty and they will keep in the fridge for several days.

Servings: 4

Preparation Time: 10 minutes

Cooking Time: 10 minutes

Total Time: 20 minutes

Ingredients

1 punnet baby plum, or other cherry tomatoes

1 pinch sea salt

1 tbsp olive oil

4 sprigs fresh thyme

Procedure

1. Preheat the oven to 200C.

2. Cut the tomatoes in half and place them cut side up on a roasting tray.

3. Drizzle with oil, scatter with salt and tuck the thyme in between evenly.

4. Roast in the hot oven until they begin to wilt; about 10 minutes.

5. Serve hot or cold, for breakfast or otherwise.

Greens with Lemon, Olive Oil and Pine Nuts

An Italian inspired side dish that goes with pretty much anything. We use Savoy cabbage for its soft texture and mild flavour but you could use spring greens, kale or any other leafy cruciferous greens. The cabbage is blanched in boiling water until just tender and then tossed in oil, lemon and toasted nuts. It is useful to blanch more cabbage than you might need; kept in the fridge with no additions it comes in handy for all manner of dishes.

Servings: 2

Preparation Time: 10 minutes

Cooking Time: 10 minutes

Total Time: 20 minutes

Ingredients

1 head Savoy cabbage, shredded

1 tbsp olive oil

2 tbsp pine nuts, toasted

1 lemon, juice only

Procedure

1. Bring a large pan of boiling water to the boil.

2. Add the cabbage and cook until tender; about 10 to 15 minutes, or less if you prefer it crisp.

3. Drain the cabbage, reserving the water for soup or stock if you wish, and toss with the lemon, oil and pinenuts.

4. Serve hot.

Roast Mediterranean Vegetables

RECIPE

Another great Paleo staple as they can be cooked in quantity, keep in the fridge well and can be enjoyed hot or cold. Served as a side dish in our plan, as well as forming the basis of two lunch meals, these roasted vegetables are easy to make and go well with so many other foods. Cutting layered vegetables such as fennel and onions with their root still intact prevents them from collapsing in the oven.

Servings: 4

Preparation Time: 20 minutes

Cooking Time: 45 minutes

Total Time: 1 hour and 5 minutes

Ingredients

2 courgettes, cut into large chunks

1 aubergine, cut in 1 inch cubes

2 red onion, quartered with root intact

1 red pepper, cut into 1 inch squares

2 bulbs young fennel, cut into 6 with root intact

2 tbsp extra virgin olive oil

1 pinch sea salt

1 tsp freshly-ground black pepper

2 sprigs fresh thyme

6 cloves garlic, still in skins

Procedure

1. Preheat the oven to 200C.

2. Place everything on a large baking tray and toss to coat thoroughly in oil.

3. Cook in the oven for about 30 minutes until the vegetables are tender and brown but not too soft. Turn occasionally with a spatula so that they cook evenly.

4. Remove from the oven and serve hot or cold.

Root Mash with Paprika and Fennel Seed

A great alternative to potatoes, full of sweet earthy flavours and far more goodness. Choose whichever varieties of roots are available and try to get as broad a range as possible. You can also serve single root mash, or sweet potato mash. Try often overlooked ingredients such as celeriac and salsify, and experiment with different flavoured oils or herbs.

Servings: 2

Preparation Time: 10 minutes

Cooking Time: 30 minutes

Total Time: 40 minutes

Ingredients

150g carrots, diced

150g parsnip, diced

150g swede, diced

1 tsp sea salt

2 tbsp olive oil

1 tsp paprika

1 tsp fennel seeds

Procedure

1. Place all the roots in a pan of salted water and bring to the boil.

2. Cook for about 20 minutes or until the roots are soft.

3. Drain, put the roots back into the pan and cover with a piece of kitchen paper to absorb excess water.

4. Put the paprika, oil and fennel into a small saucepan and heat together for a few minutes. Strain out the fennel seeds.

5. Mash the roots until soft and fluffy and serve hot with the scented oil drizzled over.

Spinach and Sweet Potato Curry

Sometimes you just need more starchy carbs than usual and this spicy side dish goes perfectly with the Tandoori Chicken. Very simple and quick to make, the dish makes the use of fresh flavours rather than a long list of spices and the flavours are spectacular. Spinach alongside the sweet potato not only brings it closer to the well-known Indian dish but adds vital nutrients to the starchy carbs.

Servings: 2

Preparation Time: 15 minutes

Cooking Time: 20 minutes

Total Time: 35 minutes

Ingredients

1 tbsp coconut oil

4 medium sweet potatoes, peeled and diced

100g baby spinach leaves

2 cloves garlic, crushed

2 inches ginger, grated

2 red chillies, finely chopped

2 tbsp fresh coriander, chopped

1 tsp cumin seeds

1 squeeze fresh lemon juice

1 pinch sea salt

Procedure

1. Boil the sweet potato in a large pan of water until tender; roughly 20 minutes.

2. Heat the coconut oil in a frying pan and add the cumin, ginger, garlic and chillies.

3. Add the sweet potato, salt, and spinach, stirring until the spinach has wilted and the sweet potato is bathed in spices; take care not to let it burn.

4. Add the coriander and a drop of lemon juice before serving hot.

Cauliflower Couscous

Far from being one of those awful Paleo substitutions, Cauliflower Couscous actually originates from the kitchen of the great chef Ferran Adria. A useful addition to Paleo cookery, Cauliflower Couscous lends its fairly neutral flavour and slightly chewy texture as a decent stand in for grains. Here we mix the cauliflower with almonds, mint and pomegranate seeds to make an excellent accompaniment to our cumin lamb chops but you could leave it plain or add any bits that you wish. It would suit a little chopped crispy bacon really well but then again what wouldn't?

Servings: 2

Preparation Time: 10 minutes

Cooking Time: 10 minutes

Total Time: 20 minutes

Ingredients

1 head cauliflower, grated or blitzed in processor

2 tbsp coconut oil

1 small bunch mint

2 tbsp flaked almonds

1 pinch sea salt

$^1/_2$ pomegranate, seeds only

Procedure

1. Blitz the cauliflower in a food processor or grate it so it resembles small grains. Remove any large uneven bits.

2. Heat the coconut oil in a large frying pan and add the grated cauliflower with a good pinch of salt.

3. Stir fry slowly until the cauliflower is tender; about 8-10 minutes.

4. Stir through the flaked almonds, mint and pomegranate seeds to serve.

EXTRAS

Basic Tomato Sauce

This basic recipe is best cooked for a few hours to create a slick and glossy tomato sauce full of flavour. Used as the base of other recipes it is a good way to inject flavour into a midweek supper without resorting to ready-made jars. Fresh herbs work best, especially if you have a few woody herbs growing outside, but dried will be just fine if it is all that you have. Woody herbs such as thyme, rosemary and bay freeze particularly well so if you buy a large bag just pop it straight into the freezer and use as required.

Servings: 6

Preparation Time: 5 minutes

Cooking Time: 2 hours

Total Time: 2 hours and 5 minutes

Ingredients

800g chopped tinned tomatoes

4 tbsp olive oil

1 tsp sea salt

1 bay leaf

2 sprigs thyme

1 sprig rosemary

1 head garlic, cut in half horizontally

Procedure

1. Place a large saucepan over a low heat and add all of the ingredients.

2. Using the empty tin, measure out the same amount of water and add to the pan.

3. Leave the sauce alone, giving it the occasional stir, until it is thick and glossy. The lower and slower it cooks, the better it will be.

4. Once done, fish out the stalks and bits before leaving to cool and using as required.

Chicken Stock

Using the bones from a roast chicken to make stock not only proves value for money in providing the means for another meal, but chicken stock is a great way of adding flavour and nutrients to a meal. Use it for making soup, cooking vegetables or making sauces; it will liven up your cooking no end.

It is always worth having cold roast chicken in the fridge for an impromptu salad when you are too tired or hungry to cook; extra bones for extra stock. You don't need to add carrots, onions, bay leaves to the stock pot, although you can if you wish. The flavour of the chicken is enough in itself and doesn't muddy other flavours with an overpowering stock. A good stock, made from decent bones, will turn to jelly in the fridge. In fact a cheap chicken from a battery hen will often make stock that refuses to set; a sure sign of immature, mineral deficient bones.

Servings: 6

Preparation Time: 10 minutes

Cooking Time: 1 hour and 30 minutes

Total Time: 1 hour and 40 minutes

Ingredients

2 small leftover chicken carcasses (cooked)

1.5 litres water

Procedure

1. You will get better stock if you chop the carcass and the long bones in half first.

2. Lay them in a large pan, preferably one with more height than girth, and cover with cold water by a few inches.

3. Bring the pot slowly to a simmer, skimming off any scum that appears on top of the liquid.

4. Keep the stock at a gentle simmer; cooking it too rapidly makes a greasy, bitter, cloudy stock.

5. Once reduced by about half, remove all bones (strain if you can) and leave to cool completely before keeping in the fridge for up to 3 days.

DESSERTS

Baked Banana
and Chocolate

A smooth and comforting dessert of banana and chocolate to satisfy a sweet tooth after a meal. You can add nuts if you wish, or flaked coconut, but without these added textures the dish is sublimely soft; exactly what you might need.

Servings: 2

Preparation Time: 5 minutes

Cooking Time: 15 minutes

Total Time: 20 minutes

Ingredients

2 bananas, unpeeled

50g dark chocolate, chopped

Procedure

1. Split the banana down the centre and stuff with chocolate.

2. Wrap in foil and bake in a hot oven until the chocolate has melted.

3. Unwrap and eat from the skin with a teaspoon.

Banana, Coconut and Almond Ice Cream

RECIPE

This is a quick, and surprisingly delicious, dessert. Keep chunks of frozen banana in the freezer so that you can whip up this treat at the end of a meal if you feel like something sweet. Try not to eat dessert each day; instead get into the habit of choosing fresh fruit or not sweetening the palate at all. If you make your own coconut milk with blocks of coconut cream you can make it really thick and creamy.

Servings: 2

Preparation Time: 5 minutes

Cooking Time: 5 minutes

Inactive Time: 1 hour

Total Time: 1 hour and 10 minutes

Ingredients

2 bananas, chopped and frozen

1 pinch ground cardamom (optional)

2 tbsp raw almonds

50ml coconut milk

Procedure

1. Blitz all of the ingredients in a processor until smooth.

2. Eat at once as it melts quickly.

Apple and Cinnamon Crunch

A warm apple dish, perfect for breakfast or dessert. Use any nuts for the topping; walnuts and brazil nuts are particularly nutritious whilst macadamia nuts are mellow and luxurious. Make extra and keep it in the fridge to eat if you wish.

Servings: 2

Preparation Time: 10 minutes

Cooking Time: 5 minutes

Total Time: 15 minutes

Ingredients

4 apples, cored and cut into wedges

1 tbsp coconut oil

1 tsp cinnamon

1 pinch nutmeg

2 tbsp almonds, roughly chopped

Procedure

1. Heat the oil in a frying pan and add the apple wedges. Toss to coat in oil and cook gently for a few minutes.

2. Sprinkle with cinnamon and nutmeg and continue cooking until soft and browned.

3. Serve hot or cold, topped with the chopped nuts.

Coconut Hot Chocolate

Melted chocolate with hot creamy coconut milk makes a soothing drink for after a meal or at the end of a day. It's quite good in bed with the Sunday papers too. Add extra coconut cream for a thicker drink. Limit consumption of such treats as even dark chocolate contains sugar; it also contains a fair amount of caffeine. But we all deserve a treat!

Servings: 2

Cooking Time: 5 minutes

Total Time: 5 minutes

Ingredients

50g dark chocolate

200ml coconut milk

Procedure

1. Stir the ingredients together in a small saucepan over a low heat until the chocolate and coconut cream have melted.

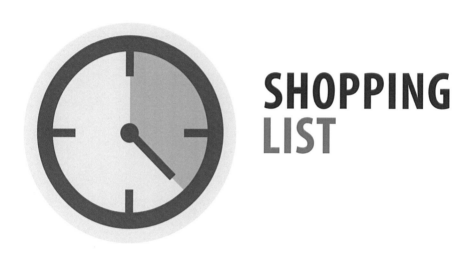

SHOPPING
LIST

Shopping List

Fat and oils	Lard, dripping or goose fat Extra virgin olive oil	Walnut oil Coconut oil	
Meat and Fish	Sausages 6 Bacon rashers 12 Smoked salmon 100g Fish fillets 400g	Smoked mackerel fillets 2 Lamb chops 4 Turkey breast steaks 700g Brisket or silverside joint 750g	Sirloin steaks 2 Chickens, small whole 4
Eggs	3 dozen		
Vegetables	Red peppers 4 Onions 5 Mushrooms, family pack Avocado 4 Baby spinach 350g Red onion 3 Large tomatoes 6 Bag of mixed salad leaves 1 Cucumber 1/2 Spring onions 2 bunches	Cherry tomatoes 1 punnet Romaine lettuce hearts 2 Savoy cabbage 1 Courgette 2 Aubergine 1 Leeks 2 Parsnips 8 Red cabbage 1/4 Fennel bulb 3 Swede 2	Fine green beans 200g Butternut squash 1 Carrots 9 Sweet potatoes 4 Cauliflower 1 Garlic bulbs 3 Red chilli pepper 10 Shallots 4
Fruit	Pomegranate 1 Apples 8	Bananas 4 Lemons 4	Limes 2
Fresh Herbs	Fresh parsley, small bunch 2 Fresh thyme, small bunch 1 Fresh dill, small bunch 1 Bay leaves 3	Fresh coriander, small bunch 2 Lemongrass 4 Large piece fresh ginger 1 Green finger chillies 4	Fresh basil, small bunch 2 Fresh mint, small bunch 2 Fresh rosemary, small bunch 1 Fresh sage leaves, small bunch 1
Chicken Stock	(bought or made fresh - see recipe) 700ml		
Dried Herbs	Black peppercorns (for grinding) Paprika Smoked paprika Maldon sea salt	Ground cumin Ground coriander Lime leaves (dried) Ground fenugreek Ground cloves	Green cardamom Fennel seeds Cinnamon ground Nutmeg whole
Store Cupboard	Coconut milk 800ml Balsamic vinegar Dijon mustard Anchovies, small tin 1 Dark chocolate 100g	Chopped tomatoes 2 tins Marinated artichokes (olive oil) 1 jar Kalamata olives 400g Pine nuts, small pack	Walnuts, small pack Flaked almonds, small pack Whole almonds, large pack Sesame seeds 100g

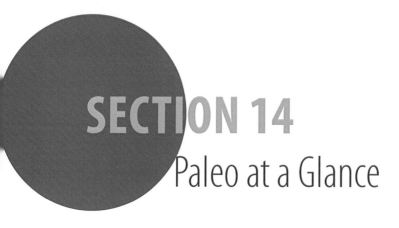

SECTION 14
Paleo at a Glance

THESE FOODS ARE NOT TO BE EATEN

DAIRY

Any dairy including (but not limited to):

- Butter
- Buttermilk
- Cheese
- Cottage cheese
- Cream
- Ice cream
- Milk
- Powdered milk
- Yoghurt

GRAINS

Any grains including (but not limited to):

- Amaranth
- Barley
- Buckwheat
- Corn
- Millet
- Oats
- Quinoa
- Rice
- Rye
- Sorghum
- Spelt
- Wheat
- Wild rice

LEGUMES

Any beans including (but not limited to):

- Adzuki beans
- Black beans
- Black eyed beans
- Chick peas
- Lentils
- Lima beans
- Mung beans
- Navy beans
- Peanuts
- Pinto beans
- Red beans
- Soy beans

SWEETENERS

Any man made sweetener (but not limited to):

- Brown sugar
- Maple syrup
- Refined honey
- Sugar cane
- White sugar

OILS

All hydrogenated refined oils including (but not limited to):

- Vegetable oil
- Sunflower
- Peanut
- Corn
- Safflower
- Soya
- Cottonseed

THESE FOODS CAN BE EATEN FREELY

VEGETABLES

All vegetables including (but not limited to):

- Artichoke, globe
- Artichoke, Jerusalem
- Asparagus
- Avocado
- Beetroot
- Aubergine
- Bok Choy
- Broccoli
- Brussels sprouts
- Cabbage
- Carrot
- Cauliflower
- Celeriac
- Celery
- Chicory
- Cucumber
- Endive
- Fennel
- Green beans
- Kale
- Kohlrabi
- Leek
- Lettuce
- Mushroom
- Okra
- Onion
- Parsnip
- Peas
- Pepper
- Sweet potato
- Pumpkin
- Radicchio
- Radish
- Rocket
- Romaine Lettuce
- Salsify
- Shallot
- Spinach
- Squash
- Swiss Chard
- Tomatillo
- Tomato
- Turnip
- Water chestnut
- Watercress

HERBS

All herbs including (but not limited to):

- Chives
- Coriander
- Dill
- Garlic
- Ginger
- Parsley
- Chilli
- Mint
- Basil
- Tarragon
- Lemongrass

FRUITS

All fruit including (but not limited to):

- Apple
- Banana
- Blackberry
- Blueberry
- Grape
- Fig
- Guava
- Lychee
- Mango
- Melon
- Papaya
- Passion Fruit
- Peach
- Plum
- Nectarine
- Pear
- Persimmon
- Pineapple
- Pomegranate
- Raspberry
- Rhubarb
- Strawberries
- Watermelon

MEAT

All unprocessed meats including (but not limited to):

- Bacon
- Beef
- Bison
- Gluten free sausages
- Goat
- Lamb
- Nitrate free salamis
- Organ meats (offal)
- Ostrich
- Pork
- Veal

POULTRY AND GAME

All Poultry and Game including (but not limited to):

- Chicken
- Duck
- Pheasant
- Pigeon
- Quail
- Rabbit
- Turkey
- Venison

EGGS

All eggs including (but not limited to):

- Hen
- Duck
- Quail

SEAFOOD

All seafood including (but not limited to):

- Mackerel
- Prawns
- Salmon
- Sardines
- Shellfish
- Tuna
- White fish (cod/haddock/ sea-bass/ monkfish etc)

NUTS AND SEEDS

All nuts and seeds including (but not limited to):

- Almonds
- Brazil
- Cashews
- Chestnuts
- Hazelnuts
- Macadamias
- Nut butters
- Pine nuts
- Pistachios
- Sesame seeds
- Sunflower seeds

FATS AND OILS

- Beef dripping
- Coconut oil
- Duck fat
- Olive oil
- Goose fat
- Hazelnut oil
- Lard
- Macadamia oil
- Walnut oil
- Avocado Oil
- Ghee

DRINKS

- Water
- Vegetable Juices

THESE FOODS CAN BE ENOYED IN MODERATION

MODERATION

- Coffee
- Dark chocolate
- Dried fruit
- Alcohol
- Raw honey
- Tea
- Fruit juice (freshly made)
- Organic Maple Syrup

Additional Books

We hope that you have enjoyed Introduction to Paleo. If you wanted to continue your Paleo journey we have three additional books to help you on your way.

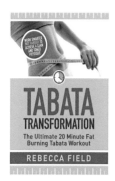

Tabata Transformation

Tabata involves short but intensive workouts designed to maximise fat loss and make you leaner and stronger in only 20 minutes. Incorporating short bursts of activity into your exercise regime is the most efficient way to burn fat and improve stamina and overall fitness levels. Tabata Transformation provides 12 weeks of varied workouts suitable for gym or home use with minimal equipment needed. We have provided illustrations of every exercise making the workouts easy to follow.

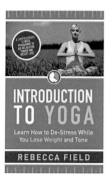

Introduction to Yoga

Yoga not only promotes relaxation and calm but provides a great allover workout; perfect for toning and posture. Learning how to effectively deal with stress will provide you with the tools you need to face life head on. Contains 12 weeks of Yoga exercises for all abilities in a variety of challenging and fun workouts to complete at home or in the gym. Illustrations have been provided so every Yoga position is clearly set out.

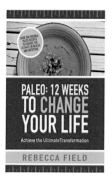

Paleo: 12 Weeks to Change Your Life

Our 12 Week Programme follows on from "Introduction to Paleo" and provides you with all the information that you need to continue your Paleo journey and achieve a truly healthy and sustainable lifestyle. With over 200 original recipes, weekly meal planners and specific shopping lists you will have all the tools you need to ensure that you adopt a healthy approach to eating even after the programme has come to an end.

All books are available for purchase from the Paleo Diet and Fitness website at www.paleodietandfitness.co.uk